W9-BVM-507

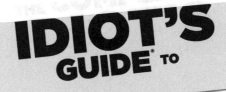

THE COMPLETE
IDIOT'S GUIDE® TO

Digestive Health

by Dustin Garth James, M.D., with Liz Scott

THOMPSON PUBLIC LIBRARY
934 RIVERSIDE DRIVE
N. GROSVENORDALE, CT 06255

SEP 2 9 2010

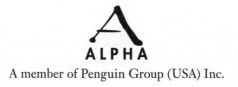

A
ALPHA

A member of Penguin Group (USA) Inc.

ALPHA BOOKS

Published by the Penguin Group

Penguin Group (USA) Inc., 375 Hudson Street, New York, New York 10014, USA

Penguin Group (Canada), 90 Eglinton Avenue East, Suite 700, Toronto, Ontario M4P 2Y3, Canada (a division of Pearson Penguin Canada Inc.)

Penguin Books Ltd., 80 Strand, London WC2R 0RL, England

Penguin Ireland, 25 St. Stephen's Green, Dublin 2, Ireland (a division of Penguin Books Ltd.)

Penguin Group (Australia), 250 Camberwell Road, Camberwell, Victoria 3124, Australia (a division of Pearson Australia Group Pty. Ltd.)

Penguin Books India Pvt. Ltd., 11 Community Centre, Panchsheel Park, New Delhi—110 017, India

Penguin Group (NZ), 67 Apollo Drive, Rosedale, North Shore, Auckland 1311, New Zealand (a division of Pearson New Zealand Ltd.)

Penguin Books (South Africa) (Pty.) Ltd., 24 Sturdee Avenue, Rosebank, Johannesburg 2196, South Africa

Penguin Books Ltd., Registered Offices: 80 Strand, London WC2R 0RL, England

Copyright © 2010 by Dustin Garth James, M.D., and Liz Scott

All rights reserved. No part of this book shall be reproduced, stored in a retrieval system, or transmitted by any means, electronic, mechanical, photocopying, recording, or otherwise, without written permission from the publisher. No patent liability is assumed with respect to the use of the information contained herein. Although every precaution has been taken in the preparation of this book, the publisher and authors assume no responsibility for errors or omissions. Neither is any liability assumed for damages resulting from the use of information contained herein. For information, address Alpha Books, 800 East 96th Street, Indianapolis, IN 46240.

THE COMPLETE IDIOT'S GUIDE TO and Design are registered trademarks of Penguin Group (USA) Inc.

International Standard Book Number: 978-1-59257-984-6
Library of Congress Catalog Card Number: 2009937005

12   11   10   8   7   6   5   4   3   2   1

Interpretation of the printing code: The rightmost number of the first series of numbers is the year of the book's printing; the rightmost number of the second series of numbers is the number of the book's printing. For example, a printing code of 10-1 shows that the first printing occurred in 2010.

Printed in the United States of America

Note: This publication contains the opinions and ideas of its authors. It is intended to provide helpful and informative material on the subject matter covered. It is sold with the understanding that the authors and publisher are not engaged in rendering professional services in the book. If the reader requires personal assistance or advice, a competent professional should be consulted.

The authors and publisher specifically disclaim any responsibility for any liability, loss, or risk, personal or otherwise, which is incurred as a consequence, directly or indirectly, of the use and application of any of the contents of this book.

Most Alpha books are available at special quantity discounts for bulk purchases for sales promotions, premiums, fund-raising, or educational use. Special books, or book excerpts, can also be created to fit specific needs.

For details, write: Special Markets, Alpha Books, 375 Hudson Street, New York, NY 10014.

Publisher: *Marie Butler-Knight*

Associate Publisher: *Mike Sanders*

Senior Managing Editor: *Billy Fields*

Senior Acquisitions Editor: *Paul Dinas*

Development Editor: *Frank Coffin*

Production Editor: *Kayla Dugger*

Copy Editor: *Amy Lepore*

Cover Designer: *William Thomas*

Book Designers: *William Thomas, Rebecca Batchelor*

Indexer: *Heather McNeill*

Layout: *Brian Massey*

Proofreader: *Laura Caddell*

In memory of Ray Clouse, M.D. His contributions to the understanding of gastrointestinal disease will never be forgotten.

Contents

Appendixes

Introduction

If you're interested in learning all about your digestive health, you've come to the right place. In this book, you'll find all you need to know about the inner workings of your digestive system, what might happen when things go awry, and how to keep you and your family in great digestive health. The subject is a big one, but we think we've narrowed it down to its essential information and covered just about every possible question you might have. From "Why do we burp?" to "How is Crohn's disease treated?"—you'll be quite the know-it-all after reading this guide.

Maybe you're particularly interested in a specific topic such as irritable bowel syndrome or how your colon conducts its business. You'll find what you want to know and more. Because we've created a comprehensive guide to all things digestive, you'll no doubt be picking up this book again and again for quick, clear answers to nagging questions or for a solid rundown of a particular disease and its diagnosis and treatment. The more you know about your digestive health, the better off you will be in the long run. It's pretty interesting stuff, too, and quite amazing the way the whole gastrointestinal system comes together to perform for us day after day.

Well, it's time to begin your journey toward great digestive health, so we won't keep you any longer. Here are just a few tidbits of information that will help you navigate through this book.

How to Use This Book

There are five parts to this book:

Part 1, Understanding the Digestive System, provides the nuts and bolts of what gastroenterology is all about, from the digestive process and its key players to your first visit with a gastroenterologist and what you might encounter.

Part 2, Upper GI Conditions and Diseases, is your detailed guide to the most common digestive disorders that occur above the colon, from acid reflux disease and its complications to gastritis, ulcers, and celiac disease.

Part 3, Lower GI Conditions and Diseases, explores the deeper bowels of the digestive process and explains disorders such as Crohn's disease, ulcerative colitis, irritable bowel syndrome, and the all-important topic of polyps and colon cancer.

Part 4, Additional Digestive-Related Conditions, discusses the potential problems that can affect some digestive side players, including the pancreas, gallbladder, and liver, while exploring the possible reasons for many tummy upsets such as viruses, bacteria, and parasites.

Part 5, Maintaining Good Digestive Health, explains how a healthy diet and lifestyle can keep you in good stead, while also discussing common food allergies, restricted diets, and natural and complementary approaches to many digestive conditions.

Extras

You'll come across many boxed notes throughout the book that provide some additional information. Watch for these:

DEFINITION

Here you'll find explanations of medical terminology and some other tricky digestive jargon.

TUMMY TIP

These provide advice and hints on a variety of digestive matters.

GULP!

Specific health warnings and alerts are found here, so be sure to check them out.

GI DIDN'T KNOW!

These contain a wealth of interesting facts, figures, and amusing trivia for your reading pleasure.

Acknowledgments

From Dustin:

Great thanks to Liz, the staff and physicians at Midwest Gastroenterology, and all the people at Alpha Books. Thanks also to my parents, Rich and Nancy, and the rest of the family, including Mandy, Andrew, Joshie, Emily, and my wonderful wife, Helen.

From Liz:

Thanks to everyone at Alpha Books, especially Paul Dinas, who deserves a medal for patience. Thank you also to Marilyn Allen, Coleen O'Shea, Larry Chilnick, Jennifer Pruden, Jim, Anna, and Connie for their support and help. Thank you "Baby" for sharing your angelic presence with me for 19 years, and thank you "Bella" for helping me heal.

Trademarks

All terms mentioned in this book that are known to be or are suspected of being trademarks or service marks have been appropriately capitalized. Alpha Books and Penguin Group (USA) Inc. cannot attest to the accuracy of this information. Use of a term in this book should not be regarded as affecting the validity of any trademark or service mark.

Understanding the Digestive System

Before you begin to improve and maintain your digestive health, you'll need to know a bit about your body's digestive system. How exactly does it work? What are the players involved? How does digestion relate to the body's other systems and contribute to overall health? In Part 1, we'll take an up-close-and-personal look at the digestive process from beginning to end.

We'll also go over some very common digestive symptoms and determine when they are serious enough that you should seek medical advice. Speaking of medical advice, you'll meet and get to know the doc who makes digestion his life's work—the gastroenterologist. We'll lay out everything you need to know about your first visit, and you'll also get a great primer on the myriad tests your doctor has at his or her disposal to sort out any digestive issues you may have. So let's take the first step to digestive health—understanding your digestive system.

Digestion and Your Health

In This Chapter

- Digesting basic health facts
- Evaluating your elimination habits
- Understanding vital connections and risks

A healthy digestive system is as important to your overall health as a healthy heart, healthy bones, and the health of other parts of the body. In fact, the state of your digestive health can affect the level of wellness you experience in your other body systems. When running smoothly, we hardly notice the inner workings of our digestive organs, but when problems arise, we may not only have a bad "gut feeling." We might experience any number of symptoms from our heads down to our toes.

The main job of our digestive system is processing the food we eat to obtain energy and absorb nutrients. Without proper energy and nutrition, we would find it difficult to accomplish just about any daily activity from walking to thinking. Even our sleep could be disrupted. But when the digestive system is doing its job correctly, our bodies can carry out normal activities with general ease—barring any other physical ailments, of course. Healthy digestion usually indicates pretty good overall health.

Mind you, even healthy people with good digestion experience the occasional belch or periodic bout of indigestion. Many common digestive symptoms such as these are simply a sign of the system at work. In Chapter 3, we'll examine these symptoms in more detail and help you determine whether they warrant further attention. For the most part, however, if you are relatively symptom free and your weight is at an acceptable level, your digestive system is getting the job done.

Rising Concerns

In spite of the ease with which our bodies normally conduct digestive business, Americans today are experiencing more gastrointestinal (GI) problems than ever before. Why this is the case has been the subject of much speculation, but for the most part, the bigger we get as a society (pound-wise), the greater our chances seem to be for developing digestive disorders. Obesity has been implicated in the rise of diseases like acid reflux and fatty liver, not to mention the near national epidemic of heart disease and diabetes we are seeing. There is also evidence that many of the foods we eat (or don't eat, for that matter) play significant roles in the rise of digestive diseases.

GI DIDN'T KNOW!

The digestive tract handles about 20,000 pounds of solid food during the average lifetime.

As we live longer, there is also greater room for natural wear and tear. Polyps may form in the colon or inflammation can occur in the esophagus simply from a long life. Conditions such as these, if left untreated, may give rise to further complications, including severe organ damage or even cancer.

The Pitfalls of Progress

Early humans who hunted and gathered their food supply probably never developed diseases such as irritable bowel syndrome (IBS) or pancreatitis. Their unprocessed and varied diet, as well as an enormous amount of daily exercise, no doubt kept them svelte and healthy. With the introduction of grain agriculture and the industrialized milling that stripped grain of vitamins, minerals, and most of its fiber, we began a downward spiral of poor eating habits. Add a sedentary lifestyle, along with smoking, drinking, and stress, and you have a recipe for poor digestive health. With all the progress we have seen as a modern society, the current average American diet and lifestyle, when it comes to maintaining digestive health, is pretty much the pits.

GI DIDN'T KNOW!

According to the latest statistics from the National Digestive Diseases Information Clearinghouse (NDDIC), 14 percent of all hospital diagnostic and therapeutic procedures are for digestive diseases.

Some Gut-Wrenching Statistics

Consider the fact that nearly half (46 percent) of all Americans say digestive problems affect their lives on a daily basis. That's a rather high percentage for a civilized and medically advanced nation with the freedom to make healthy choices. Although 80 percent feel it's important to improve their digestive health, most are doing little about it. In fact, until we are faced with some uncomfortable symptoms such as heartburn or constipation, most of us pay little attention to the digestive process and the importance of keeping our digestive health in check.

TUMMY TIP

Don't be embarrassed to discuss digestive issues with your health-care provider during routine visits. Always ask questions about any concerns you may have.

Understanding how your body processes food, learning about healthy eating, and monitoring your digestive health with your doctor through periodic screening will go a long way toward reducing your chances of being in the unfortunate group of Americans who cope with digestive issues every day. Early detection, advanced technology, and even the means to cure diseases that were once incurable have revolutionized the field of *gastroenterology*. Along with our growing awareness of the value in prevention and maintenance of digestive health, we may just be on a healthier path after all. If knowledge is power, educating yourself about all things digestive will give you the wellness edge you need.

DEFINITION

Gastroenterology is a specialized field of medicine concerned with the function and disorders of the digestive system.

The Process of Elimination

We know that we consume food in order to glean valuable nutrients and energy, but unless we have x-ray eyes, we may not be able to visualize easily the process occurring within our bodies. In essence, all that we see is what goes in one end and comes out the other. Although it's clearly much more appetizing to watch our food go down the hatch, keeping an eye on the quality of what is being eliminated can tell us a lot about how things are functioning inside.

GULP!

Don't be alarmed if food actually makes an appearance in your stool. It is normal for high-fiber foods such as corn, beans, seeds, and nuts to occasionally pass undigested.

The ideal bowel movement is medium brown in color, measures between 4 and 8 inches in length, and is the consistency of toothpaste. It should leave the body without effort and be relatively free of odor and gas. Occasional variations can occur for any number of reasons, such as the food or drink we have consumed or medicines we are taking, but in general, your solid waste should be similar to this description, indicating a healthy elimination process.

Color Me Concerned

Of all the types of visual changes to your stool that can occur, alterations in color are often the ones that prompt concern. Here are a few explanations for possible variations in color:

Gray or pale stool could indicate decreased bile output. Initially, bile, an important fluid produced by the liver to aid digestion, turns stool a hue of green. Then bacteria present in the colon turn the green to brown, the color we normally associate with stool. Use of antacids may also cause light-colored stool.

Green stool may mean that food is passing through the digestive tract faster than normal and the bacteria have not had a chance to make a color change to brown. Iron supplements also contribute to a dark green hue, sometimes even black.

Yellow stool, like pale stool, could also indicate a decrease in bile or that food may be passing too quickly through the body. People with acid reflux disease might produce yellow-colored stool.

Black stool can indicate upper digestive tract bleeding. A "tarry" and quite smelly black stool, also referred to as melena, is the result of bacteria digesting blood that is present. Bismuth, found in Pepto-Bismol and similar products, or dark foods such as licorice, however, can also cause black coloration.

GULP!

Unexplained deep red- or black-colored stools should prompt an immediate visit to your doctor. Be aware, however, that the presence of blood is not always visible; therefore, it's equally important to speak with your doctor about any other changes or abnormalities you notice in your stool.

Red stool may indicate bleeding from any area of the digestive tract or the presence of hemorrhoids or fissures. Eating beets or foods prepared with red food coloring, such as red velvet cake, can also cause red stool.

High and Low Frequency

The frequency of bowel movements, or "regularity," is a subject we hear a lot about with differing opinions. Is it necessary to have a movement every day? How about every other day? The truth is that as long as you are symptom free—meaning no pain or discomfort and without excess bloating, heartburn, or other sensations—a movement every three or four days may be normal for you. For someone else, three or four movements a day could be considered normal. Be aware that frequency can often be temporarily disrupted by a change in activity such as traveling or exercise, as well as events such as menstruation or surgery. Unless these occasional irregularities are accompanied by other symptoms, they're generally not something to worry about. A persistent change in bowel habits, however, requires an immediate evaluation.

> **TUMMY TIP**
>
> Traveling by air is particularly dehydrating due to dry air in the cabin and often results in temporary "irregularity," particularly constipation. Always drink plenty of water during your flight and avoid alcohol and caffeine, which will only dehydrate you further.

Your Personal Plumbing System

When it comes to visualizing the inner workings of your digestive system, a little knowledge about plumbing can help. Your *alimentary canal* is really nothing more than an intricate connection of pipes and fixtures like home plumbing. With the assistance of strategically placed traps, valves, and pumps, these passages wind their way up, down, and around the inner walls, working together to process, deliver, and eliminate. If the quality of any of the fixtures is in question or a valve or other mechanism isn't functioning properly, it can wreak havoc with the entire system.

> **DEFINITION**
>
> The **alimentary canal** is another name for the GI or digestive tract.

Your inner plumbing system, if stretched out from beginning to end, measures between 25 and 30 feet long. So there is definitely room for potential problems and glitches to occur. It's quite amazing when you think about it. The vast majority of the time, your digestive system just carries on doing its job, 24/7, without a hitch. Most household plumbing can't match that success rate. But when something goes wrong, we definitely know it. So, as with household plumbing, it's helpful to become acquainted with the nature of the problems you may confront. In simple terms, digestive disorders fall into one of two categories: organic or functional.

Am I Dysfunctional?

Let's suppose your kitchen sink is clogged. There's a good chance that something you've put down the drain is causing a blockage in the pipe, disrupting the flow of water. As far as you know, there's nothing wrong with the pipes themselves. You've had them checked recently, and you may not even know what caused the blockage in the first place, but there it is. Your kitchen plumbing is experiencing a functional disorder. There is no structural explanation, and the cause is unknown.

GI DIDN'T KNOW!

Not long ago, functional disorders were dismissed as mental or imaginary. Thankfully, we now accept that a functional disorder simply means the cause is unknown.

To deal with the problem, you pour some commercial declogging liquid in the sink drain, and after an allotted amount of time, it dissolves and moves whatever is clogging the pipe. Later that day, you happen to remember that you inadvertently threw some potato peelings down the drain and that the last time you did so, the drain also clogged. You pledge that from now on, potato peelings will be put only in the trash can, and as a result, your kitchen pipes cease clogging.

Just like your kitchen plumbing, the cause of functional digestive disorders can often be difficult to ascertain. Disorders such as IBS and functional *dyspepsia* fall into this category. Once your doctor has determined that there is no organic or structural cause for your symptoms, however, he or she will probably make recommendations, called symptomatic therapy, for temporary relief (declogging liquid) and dietary alterations (no more potato peels). It is always a good idea to keep a food and symptom diary when you are experiencing persistent problems such as constipation or diarrhea. The diary may help uncover a connection between what you are eating and the symptoms you are experiencing. By eliminating certain habits or foods from your diet, your symptoms may very well subside or disappear.

DEFINITION

Dyspepsia is the general medical term for indigestion and has been poetically called "the remorse of a guilty stomach."

How Are Your Pipes?

Returning to the kitchen analogy, let's suppose that you haven't had your plumbing checked in ages and that an annoying and continual clogging of the sink drain has prompted you to call in the plumber. He gets out his wrench and flashlight and decides to take a closer look at that pipe under the sink. What he finds isn't pretty. The inside of the pipe is corroded and uneven, causing just about anything that goes down the drain to get stuck and create a clog. As opposed to a functional problem, he's found an organic one, clearly caused by structural damage. Chances are a new pipe and the writing of a large check loom on your horizon.

Digestively speaking, although you probably won't require pipe replacement, an abnormality or damage to a part of your digestive system indicates the presence of an organic disorder. This diseased state is most likely responsible for your symptoms, and appropriate treatment will need to be prescribed. Ailments such as ulcers or tumors fall under this category and will likely require more than a change in diet.

GI DIDN'T KNOW!

As a result of the large worldwide increase in occurrences of functional digestive disorders such as IBS, the Rome Criteria were created in 1989 by a group of international physicians. These criteria assist in defining and categorizing this often difficult-to-diagnose group of illnesses.

Whether functional or organic, chronic digestive problems are certainly not fun and could become serious if ignored. We'll be taking a much closer look at potential GI disorders and diseases later on, but for now, let's continue to explore the inner workings of your pipes.

The Brain-Belly Connection

Who hasn't felt nauseated from nervousness before public speaking? How about the sensation of a blow to the stomach after hearing a piece of shocking news? If you were told that it's in your mind, well, frankly, it is. The brain and belly are so intricately connected that not only can emotions trigger symptoms of a gastrointestinal nature, but digestive issues can also affect mood and emotion. This is because your entire digestive process is CEO'd by something called the *enteric nervous system* (*ENS*). The ENS keeps an impressive communication network running between the alimentary canal walls and your brain via the visceral nervous system and spinal cord. Think of it as an electrical monitoring system for the complex plumbing of an industrial site—except that your gut is a lot more complicated.

DEFINITION

The **enteric nervous system (ENS)** is a subdivision of the peripheral nervous system (PNS) that connects the central nervous system (CNS) to the body's limbs and organs. Sometimes called the "second brain," the ENS controls the GI system and is capable of making autonomic, or involuntary, decisions.

Pavlov's Pavlova

Remember old Pavlov's dogs that salivated when a bell rang because they associated the sound with the imminent arrival of food? That was a definite brain-belly connection at work, and if you've ever begun salivating just thinking about a delicious dessert, such as a Pavlova, you've experienced the same thing. But even more than mere saliva production can be triggered. Your stomach and intestines can begin to contract, and even digestive enzymes may start to secrete. It also makes perfect sense that just as something enticing can start the process, anxiety-producing situations and unappetizing thoughts can produce the opposite effect—nausea and a need to purge.

GI DIDN'T KNOW!

Ivan Pavlov's experiments on digestion earned him the 1904 Nobel Prize in physiology and medicine.

The Sensitive Gut

Some people are more sensitive to this remarkable connection and consequently may be predisposed to certain kinds of functional digestive disorders such as IBS. While others may appear to have "nerves of steel" or an "iron stomach," people with a sensitive gut may be particularly susceptible to stress and emotional turmoil and the adverse effect it has on their digestion. Disturbances along the brain-belly pathway, like glitches in your plumbing system, can cause both high-intensity and low-intensity symptoms. For example, a condition known as urgency-type diarrhea, which usually occurs right after a meal, is probably due to extreme ENS intensity, while bouts of bloating and constipation could be the result of very low intensity. Fortunately, we are learning more and more about the intricacies of the brain-belly connection, which will greatly help in the diagnosis and treatment of functional disorders that have previously puzzled both patients and physicians.

GULP!

In some sensitive-gut patients (including 50 percent of IBS sufferers), a condition known as visceral hypersensitivity can occur in which even a light touch to the abdomen can be excruciatingly painful.

Digestive Problems—Who's at Risk?

A poor diet and lifestyle can certainly create digestive problems for all of us, but are there some people who are at greater risk than others? Unfortunately, many *systemic diseases* can be responsible for common digestive disorders as well. In fact, more than half of all digestive problems encountered by physicians are the result of a systemic condition.

DEFINITION

Systemic diseases are disorders that affect the entire body rather than a single organ or body part. Diseases such as high blood pressure or influenza are categorized as systemic.

Common Culprits

Although there are numerous health conditions that can bring on problems with your digestion, if you suffer from any of the following disorders, your chances of developing digestive complications are definitely increased:

- Atherosclerosis (clogged arteries)
- Diabetes (types 1 and 2)
- Congestive heart failure
- Low blood pressure
- Scleroderma (skin or connective tissue diseases)
- History of stroke
- Chronic obstructive pulmonary disease (COPD)
- Thyroid problems (over- or underactive)
- Sickle cell anemia
- Lymphoma and other cancers

Sometimes GI symptoms make an appearance even before the actual systemic disease is diagnosed, so always be sure to alert your doctor to any unusual changes you notice to your individual digestive pattern. Early testing, diagnosis, and treatment can make a big difference when it comes to battling any disease.

GULP!

Patients with HIV or AIDS should always contact their doctors when digestive problems arise. Because of a compromised immune system, there is a high risk of developing complications.

Risk Reduction

Knowing you are at greater risk may be half the battle. In this way, you and your doctor can anticipate problems before they arise and can be prepared with medication recommendations. Clearly, there is an undeniably close connection between overall health and digestive health. Warding off any potential diseases, particularly if you are at higher risk than others because of personal or family history, can go a long way toward protecting your digestive health both now and in the future.

The Least You Need to Know

- The state of your digestive health influences your overall health and vice versa.
- Digestive problems can be either functional (without known cause) or organic (having structural cause).
- Some people are more susceptible to digestive disorders than others because of genetic or other risk factors.
- Everyone can benefit from understanding the digestive process and learning how to reduce the possibility of future GI problems.

Your Digestive Team Players

In This Chapter

- Understanding the digestive process
- Getting to know the major and minor players
- Learning about specific GI activities

It's time to take a closer look at the digestive process and get better acquainted with your team players. Every member of "team digestive" has a specific job to perform in order for digestion to run smoothly. Getting to know their individual duties is crucial to understanding the collective process as well as to recognizing problems that might arise. As in any team activity, if one guy fluffs off or can't perform, the whole group's effort could literally go down the tubes.

The digestive game begins in the mouth, although technically it's not considered a true member of the team. The mouth's contribution, however, is vital because it's here that the body begins to break down the food we eat with digestive juices—saliva secreted from glands located under the tongue and in the lower jaw area. There are actually two different types of saliva. One is thin and watery and moistens food; another is thick and mucouslike and acts as a lubricant to form chewed food into a ball-shaped mass called a bolus that can be swallowed. Once the "ball" is passed to the esophagus, the digestive game has officially begun.

The esophagus, stomach, small intestine, and colon—or large intestine—are the key players to watch. They'll be doing the bulk of the work, assisted by a few players on the sidelines, specifically the pancreas, gallbladder, and liver. Unlike most games, digestion can actually take anywhere from 24 to 72 hours to finish, kind of like a British cricket match, which has been described by Americans as baseball in slow motion. Still, it's quite a riveting activity to behold—digestion, that is—so let's take our seats and let the games begin!

The Esophagus

Up first is the esophagus, a narrow, muscular, stretchy tube about 10 inches in length that begins at the back of the mouth and continues down to the stomach. At its beginning is something called the pharynx—a kind of switch hitter, if you will—that receives both food and air from the mouth, although never at the same time or we'd choke. In order to prevent choking, the pharynx is assisted by a little flap called the epiglottis, which closes the entry to the trachea when food is to be directed down the esophagus and opens to allow air down the windpipe when we breathe. During swallowing, food always has the "right of way," and air passage is temporarily stopped.

> **GULP!**
>
> The main cause of choking in adults is insufficient chewing of food, but talking or laughing while eating can cause pieces of food to "go down the wrong pipe" and trigger choking.

A Short Journey

It takes only about eight or nine seconds for the bolus to travel down the esophagus. When the bolus reaches the end, it meets a muscular ring called a sphincter that opens and shuts to allow food to pass into the stomach and to keep acidic fluid and food from back-washing into the throat. If not protected by this mechanism, the delicate lining of the esophagus would quickly become inflamed or damaged, which would lead to heartburn, among other symptoms (see Chapter 5 on acid reflux disease). Fortunately, most of the time, this quick journey is completed without a hitch.

> **GI DIDN'T KNOW!**
>
> Because of the close proximity of the esophagus to vocal cords of the windpipe, people who have acid reflux often experience hoarseness and coughing as chronic symptoms.

Moving Right Along

Except for the voluntary actions of swallowing at the beginning and releasing stool at the end, all digestive movement is caused by an involuntary action called *peristalsis*. This movement of swallowed food through the digestive system is entirely under the control of the enteric nervous system (ENS) that we met in the last chapter. As the manager of the team, the ENS keeps the process moving along while we carry on with our lives, whether we are working, sleeping, or even standing on our heads. ENS management of the esophagus is relatively short lived compared to its work with other players. Still, although no actual digestion takes place there, the esophagus is instrumental in "keeping the ball rolling."

DEFINITION

Peristalsis is a series of wavelike muscle contractions that either propel food in one direction along the digestive tract or clean up the tract afterward like a stadium sweeper.

The Stomach

Once the bolus passes through the sphincter, it enters the realm of the hard-working stomach. Here the second phase of digestion takes place. The stomach sits in the upper-left side of the abdominal cavity just under the ribs, awaiting the arrival of food. When not directly participating in the digestive process, the average adult stomach is about ⅕ cup in volume, but just you wait! Once the stomach gets into the game, it can expand to an impressive size, holding more than 8 cups of food. And what it does with that food is equally impressive.

GI DIDN'T KNOW!

The stomach, like the heart, also has a pacemaker, causing muscle contractions to occur three times every minute.

Is It Soup Yet?

Over the next three hours or so, the stomach grinds, churns, and liquefies food it has received. Acid secretions assist in the breakdown and also kill many food-borne germs, while mucous coats the food and protects the lining of the stomach from the acid's intensity. Other secretions contribute as well. A substance known as pepsin breaks down proteins into smaller units, while another called lipase helps with fats. The end result is a soupy mix of half-digested glop called chyme. Most of the lipase in the body comes from the pancreas, though, and acts in the small intestine.

Ring My Bell

When the chyme is ready to be passed to the small intestine, specifically the *duodenum*, the stomach signals the pyloric sphincter, a valve located at the bottom of the stomach, to open its door. Not always the most cooperative doorman, the sphincter may refuse to open if the small intestine is busy doing other things such as processing a previous delivery of chyme. No problem. The stomach simply stores the half-digested food until the small intestine is ready.

DEFINITION

The **duodenum** is the first and smallest section of the small intestine and is the principal site where chemical digestion takes place.

The actual size of digested food that "moves" into the small intestine is quite small. Larger, nondigested items such as fiber must wait their turn, leaving at the end of the stomach's digestive cycle. Another factor affecting the passing of chyme to the small intestine is the amount of fats and/or alcohol ingested; these slow the emptying process a bit. On average, it takes about two to four hours to empty liquids and four to six hours to empty solids.

Ruminate This

Of course, if humans had the advantage that animals such as cows and sheep have, waiting on the sphincter might not be an issue. These mammals, called ruminators, actually have three fore-stomachs in their digestive team's roster. Consequently, they have the ability to regurgitate the bolus, called the "cud," and digest it again and again and again. In a similar fashion, most birds have an additional specialized stomach called a gizzard where they ingest stones that help grind food, particularly helpful when you don't have teeth. Human stomachs, on the other hand, just get one shot at this phase of digestion, so it's especially important that everything is operating in top-notch form.

The Small Intestine

When the soupy chyme makes its way past the pyloric sphincter, it's the small intestine's turn to take over. Long, narrow, and muscular, this digestive player can measure about 22 feet in length, although you'd never realize it the way it compactly coils itself like a snake within the abdominal cavity. Arguably, the small intestine is the most important part of the digestive system. Its job is to really process the chyme so that nutrients are properly digested and absorbed, and indeed, the small intestine is the site where a vast majority of nutrients are absorbed. To handle this formidable task, the small intestine is composed of three distinct and important sections—the duodenum (about 10 inches in length), the jejunum (about 8 feet in length), and the longest section called the ileum (nearly 12 feet in length).

GI DIDN'T KNOW!

In spite of its name, the small intestine is the largest human organ (except for skin) and is much longer than the large intestine. Its width, however, is not as great as that of the large intestine, and that fact is responsible for its designation as "small."

The Dynamic "Duo"

The duodenum is where secretions from the pancreas, liver, and gallbladder arrive. These liquids help to decrease the acidity content of chyme and further assist in the digestive process. Interestingly, it is believed that these acid-neutralizing liquids are the primary cause of sleepiness after a meal, as they turn blood more alkaline. In addition, various *enzymes* turn proteins into amino acids, carbohydrates into simple sugars, and fat into glycerol and fatty acid as food makes its long journey through the small intestine. This dynamic occurrence usually takes between one and four hours, depending on what we've eaten and how much water is present.

DEFINITION

Enzymes are proteins that can cause chemical changes in organic substances such as food.

Up the Villi

Once food reaches the jejunum, it's pretty much ready to be absorbed through millions of teeny, fingerlike projections called villi, which are located on the lumen, the inner surface lining of the intestinal wall. Here, villi pick up nutrients and deliver them to the bloodstream and to the liver. Nearly all nutrients are absorbed here, with a few exceptions such as iron, which the duodenum absorbs, or vitamin B_{12}, which the ileum absorbs.

After every possible nutrient has been gleaned from the traveling chyme by the jejunum, it moves on to the final section of the small intestine—the ileum. Here, a last-ditch effort is made to absorb any remaining nutrients before passing the chyme on to the large intestine, the final big player of the digestive game.

The Large Intestine

About 5 feet in length and 3 inches wide, the large intestine is the digestive team's cleanup batter. It is often simply referred to as the colon, the very first part of which is called the cecum, a pouch that connects the ileum of the small intestine to the ascending colon. The cecum is a bit wider than the rest of the colon, which continues up, over, and down the abdominal cavity, finally ending at the rectum—a short, 5-inch-long segment attached to the anal canal.

GI DIDN'T KNOW!

The colon definitely gets around. It extends up the right side of the abdomen, across the upper gut, and down your left side, accounting for the technical terms used to describe each section: ascending colon, transverse colon, and descending colon.

What's left of the chyme after the small intestine has done its job is handled by this big organ over the course of 32 hours or so. The watery mess it's been dumped with becomes solid when the colon is finished with it, after squeezing out and absorbing up to a gallon of water and more than an ounce of salt. The colon even manages to absorb a few remaining nutrients with the help of some friendly bacteria. Technically speaking, the chyme now becomes feces, containing dietary fiber, connective tissue from meat, and a few stubborn undigested nutrients. It also contains bacteria-digested bile, which provides the brown color we typically associate with feces.

Beneficial Bacteria

The colon provides a home for billions of bacterial flora, many of which have not even been identified yet, but they definitely don't live rent free. In fact, their contribution to the large intestine and your digestive health is quite commendable. In addition to assisting in wringing out every last nutrient from undigested fiber, they are responsible for manufacturing some important vitamins themselves, such as vitamin K and biotin. We'll be meeting these digestive heroes more intimately later, but for now, know that their presence is not only welcome but, in many instances, as we are learning, actually essential to overall health.

GI DIDN'T KNOW!

Studies on bacteria in the colon were prompted by the developing U.S. space program when concern arose that astronauts might pick up alien bacteria when they visited the moon.

The Buck Stops Here

The final stop for feces is the area of the large intestine called the rectum. Here, feces await elimination. A full rectum creates pressure that forces the walls of the anal canal to expand and receive fecal matter. It is then up to the valve known as the anal sphincter to open and allow the feces to pass out of the body. If for some reason we do not act on the urge to defecate, feces often return to the colon through reverse peristalsis. Delaying elimination, however, can result in hardened stool and uncomfortable constipation, so it is always prudent to heed nature's call.

TUMMY TIP

Just as delaying defecation can cause problems, forcing a bowel movement is never a good idea either, and it can lead to hemorrhoids, bleeding, or diverticulosis and diverticulitis. Only apply as much force as you would to blow your nose.

Once the bathroom flush takes place, it's pretty much "game over" as far as team digestive is concerned, although the team probably already has another round underway. Industrious and diligent, as long as you keep eating, your team will keep doing its jobs.

It's only fair to give credit to some sideline players that haven't received top billing but that are important nonetheless to the final outcome. Let's meet them briefly and discover what skills they bring to the digestive process.

The Pancreas

This glandular organ, about the size of your hand, actually plays on two teams at once—team digestive and team endocrine. The pancreas is probably best known for its role in the endocrine system, an important body system that releases hormones that communicate throughout the body to regulate metabolism, growth, and sexual development, among other things. In an endocrine capacity, the pancreas is most famous for secreting the hormone insulin, which is required to regulate the uptake of glucose from the blood and is associated with the disease of *diabetes mellitus*. The pancreas also secretes glucagon, another hormone that's instrumental in the metabolism of carbohydrates we consume.

DEFINITION

Diabetes mellitus is a disorder characterized by abnormally high blood sugar (glucose) levels, and it can be due to reduced production of insulin (type 1) or resistance to its effects (type 2). Although associated with eating, diabetes is classified as a metabolic disease and not a digestive one.

Via Ducts

When the pancreas is playing for team digestive—or working in its exocrine, as opposed to endocrine, capacity—it contributes enzymes to the process via the pancreatic duct, which drains into the duodenum of the small intestine. Hormones in the cells of the stomach and duodenum alert the pancreas to come in from the sidelines and start doing this job when food is present. The enzymes provided are important in digesting fats, proteins, and carbohydrates, but the pancreatic duct also secretes bicarbonate ions, which are alkaline and help to neutralize the acidity of the chyme after it arrives in the small intestine from the stomach.

GI DIDN'T KNOW!

Bicarbonate ions can create compounds called bicarbonate salts, the most famous of which is sodium bicarbonate, or baking soda—the main ingredient that neutralizes excess stomach acid in products such as Alka-Seltzer. Sodium bicarbonate, when combined with an acid such as vinegar, also allows baked goods to rise.

Nervous Impact

Although the pancreas and its related diseases usually fall under the study of endocrinology rather than gastroenterology, any abnormalities or disorders can have a large impact on the digestive process. For example, people who suffer from diabetes type 2 sometimes develop a condition called gastroparesis, or slow stomach emptying. This can occur as a result of chronic high levels of glucose in the blood. Over time, these levels may lead to nerve damage throughout the body, but in this case specifically to the *vagus nerve.* In severe cases, food may not only move slowly but stop moving altogether, a condition that could lead to bacterial growth or blockages in the stomach and duodenum. In addition to the exocrine role the pancreas plays, the potential for these sorts of digestive complications makes it an important, if not primary, member of the digestive team.

> **DEFINITION**
>
> The **vagus nerve,** which stretches from the brain to the abdomen, controls the movement of food from the stomach through the digestive tract and works with the ENS to regulate digestion.

The Gallbladder

Another important player that makes a significant contribution to team digestive is the gallbladder, a small, pear-shaped sac circuitously attached to the duodenum through a series of ducts called the biliary system. The gallbladder's sole job is to store bile produced by the liver. It's sort of a batboy in a sense, keeping a supply on hand for future use, although while bile is under the gallbladder's control, it becomes quite concentrated and more potent than when received from the liver. Bile, also called "gall" for obvious reasons, is necessary for the digestion of fat and is released into the duodenum along with other digestive juices previously discussed when chyme arrives in the small intestine.

Sidestepping Stones

Bile consists of a number of substances, including water, cholesterol, and salts. Occasionally, the cholesterol forms lumps in the gallbladder or bile duct. These lumps are called gallstones. A rapid breakdown of red blood cells in the body can also give way to a type of gallstone called a pigment stone. Regardless of the source, of the 20 million Americans who have them, most never even notice. But when gallstones do cause problems, it's hard not to take note. Sharp pain can occur on the right side and upper portion of the abdomen and even radiate to the back and shoulder because of a blockage or the gallbladder simply contracting after releasing bile. Serious complications can definitely happen (see Chapter 13 on gallbladder conditions), and the pain may be difficult to bear. As a result, and to avoid infection and possible pancreatitis, most people opt to have their gallbladders surgically removed after an attack, although in some instances stones can actually be dissolved or broken up.

Nonvital but Humorous

Because the gallbladder is considered to be a dispensable member of team digestive, it's often referred to as a "nonvital" organ like the spleen. The liver, which produces the bile in the first place, will still make sure that bile is released when necessary. Normally the team functions quite well without the gallbladder, but on occasion, particularly after a fat-laden meal, the gallbladder's absence may be missed as the liver attempts, sometimes unsuccessfully, to keep pace with bile demand.

> **GI DIDN'T KNOW!**
>
> All invertebrates as well as some vertebrates, including the horse, deer, llama, and rat, lack gallbladders as part of their digestive systems.

On another note, the yellow bile stored by the gallbladder has always been believed to play an important role in proper health. According to ancient physicians (and even up to the nineteenth century), bile is considered to be one of the four essential "humors" or substances of the body that, if imbalanced, were thought to cause disease and even affect one's personality. A shortage of yellow bile, according to this theory, would result in lethargy and a lack of ambition and passion, while a surplus could cause someone to become "bilious," meaning angry and mean spirited—a related meaning of "bile" that endures even today.

The Liver

Unlike the gallbladder, the liver is a vital organ with a multitude of functions (more than 500 at last count). These functions are relevant not only to the digestive system but to the entire body. Without the liver we could not survive, and frankly, as far as team digestive is concerned, it might as well throw in the towel before entering the ring. A true workhorse of a player, the liver, in addition to manufacturing bile, constantly regulates, converts, stores, processes, and filters any number of substances that we take into our bodies through what we ingest, breathe in, and absorb through the skin. It's a major job. Weighing in at between 3 and 3½ pounds, reddish-brown in color, and the average size of an American football, the liver rests (if ever!) to the right of the stomach and just below the diaphragm.

> **GULP!**
>
> The continuous filtering of harmful substances by the liver may result in serious liver disease, which can affect not only the digestive system but the entire body. In Western societies, alcohol is the most common cause of liver disease.

Team Multitasker

Remember all the little villi in the small intestine that were busily absorbing nutrients from the chyme and passing them on to the bloodstream? Well, all the blood that leaves both the stomach and small intestine must pass through the liver first. Remarkably, in its multitasking capacity, the liver actually receives blood from two sources: oxygen-rich blood from the heart's aorta through the hepatic artery, and nutrient-rich blood from the digestive tract through the hepatic portal vein. At any given time, the liver is dealing with about 13 percent of the entire body's blood—no small feat to be sure.

During this process, drugs as well as nutrients are broken down into forms we can ultimately use, while the liver simultaneously filters out any nasty stuff such as poisons, toxins, and bacteria, including things such as alcohol and air pollution. The liver then breaks down these harmful substances and releases them in one of two ways, either as a bile byproduct into the intestines for removal in feces or as a blood byproduct into the kidneys for further filtering and removal through urine. The liver also stores an excess of certain vitamins such as A, D, K, and B_{12} and produces about 80 percent of the body's cholesterol, among its myriad duties.

Organ, Heal Thyself!

If these feats aren't impressive enough for you, the liver is the only organ that can actually regenerate itself. This power is definitely a good thing because, unfortunately, there is a heck of a lot that can go wrong given all that the liver does. Liver diseases, from inflammation to cancer, are not uncommon and are frequently serious if not diagnosed early (see Chapter 14). Yet the ability of the liver to renew itself and even to grow a whole organ from as little as 25 percent of its tissue has made it possible for many liver-related diseases to be thwarted in early stages. Recent studies have shown that, unlike the regeneration of stem cells, the liver may actually repair itself through the simple regrowth of regular cells.

GI DIDN'T KNOW!

The ancient Greeks certainly knew about the regeneration of the liver. In their myth of Prometheus, the Titan who was chained to a rock as punishment for giving fire to mortals, an eagle devoured his liver (yikes!) every day, only to have it grow back to be eaten again the next day.

The Least You Need to Know

- The digestive system consists of the esophagus, stomach, small intestine, and large intestine.
- Organs such as the pancreas, gallbladder, and liver also contribute to the digestive process.
- Every part of the digestive system plays a specific role in properly processing the food we eat for energy and nutrition and eliminating waste.
- A problem with one part of the digestive system can affect another part and influence the entire process.
- Learning about the way normal digestion works helps you better understand when things go wrong.

Common Digestive Symptoms

In This Chapter

- Understanding the causes behind common digestive problems
- Discerning when problems require further attention
- Selecting a good gastroenterologist

Now that you know how a normal digestive system works, it's time to take a look at some common symptoms that can occur during the digestive process. Chances are you've experienced all of these symptoms at some time or other, and most of the time they do not warrant worry or concern. Many symptoms, such as occasional gas or constipation, can be caused simply by what we are eating (or not eating, for that matter). Although such symptoms may annoy us periodically, we needn't be alarmed or seek medical attention for minor complaints. In most cases, they are transitory and go away almost as quickly as they arrived.

That fact noted, the human digestive process is clearly complex, as we saw in the last chapter. Given the variety of activities that are underway from ingestion to elimination, it's surprising that we don't experience problems more often than we do—a real tribute to the body's innate wisdom. Still, it's always a good idea to note your experience with certain symptoms and whether they are associated with specific types of meals, activities, or times of day. All of this information will prove invaluable if you end up consulting with your doctor later.

Many disorders of the digestive system can display similar symptoms. Nausea, for example, could indicate anything from a stomach virus to hepatitis. However, it could also be caused by a non-gastrointestinal (GI) condition such as a bladder infection or be an adverse effect of medications. Similarly, your stomach ache or abdominal pain may not even be caused by a digestive issue at all but rather a condition such as a cyst on an ovary. These varying possibilities show why it is important to notice whether your specific symptom is accompanied by any other symptoms that could give your health-care provider insight as to a possible cause. This information is also important in determining appropriate tests that should be conducted. Any symptom, however, that becomes chronic or has a tendency to recur should be investigated. Some symptoms, like blood in the stool, require immediate attention. The sooner you are able to find and address the cause, the sooner you'll be back on a normal digestive track.

Burping and Belching

A burp or belch is the release of gas, mainly nitrogen and oxygen, from the esophagus or stomach, typically caused by swallowing air when we are eating or drinking. Belches are often accompanied by a recognizable burping sound and occasionally an odor of food. Belches that smell like rotten food may be caused by slow stomach emptying or a blockage of the bowel. Those with an odor akin to feces could indicate a colon blockage.

GI DIDN'T KNOW!

When cattle burp, they release an enormous amount of methane gas, which is a byproduct of their unique digestive systems and is believed to be a major contributor to the greenhouse effect of global warming.

Drinking carbonated beverages such as sodas and beer can also cause belching. In those instances, the gas that is released is carbon dioxide and comes from the drink itself. In addition, many types of food—anything from onions to chocolate—can cause you to belch, mainly because of the gases produced in the stomach during the initial stage of digestion. Other food culprits include milk, eggs, wheat, corn, soy, and citrus fruits. Many prescribed medications—such as those for diabetes, asthma, or depression—can initially cause excessive belching or result in persistent belching.

A Mere Hiccup?

The sound of a burp or belch is caused by the vibration that occurs when gas passes up through the valve called the upper esophageal sphincter. This valve is actually under conscious control, which is the reason we can often suppress a belch or force one out. Incidentally, the loudest belch on record was recorded in 2008 at

107.1 decibels, slightly louder than a chainsaw. Most burps, however, are not nearly so vocal and may even be silent, often confused with hiccups. As with belching, carbonated beverages can also induce hiccupping, but the two phenomena are quite different. Although they both involve the influx of air, hiccupping is completely involuntary and is caused by spasmodic contractions of the diaphragm.

Keeping Burps at Bay

If you are troubled by persistent burping, you need to examine not only what you are ingesting but how you are ingesting it. People who gulp down food and beverages naturally take in more air. Drinking through straws or squeeze bottles also increases the amount of air we swallow. Smokers and gum chewers can also inadvertently ingest air, and dentures that do not fit allow air to sneak through as well. Be sure to chew food slowly and thoroughly. Unexplained chronic belching could indicate a food allergy, gallbladder issue, acid reflux disease, hiatal hernia, *H. pylori* bacteria, gastritis, or slow digestion due to ulcers or other conditions. Be sure to consult your doctor, particularly if your burping is accompanied by other symptoms.

TUMMY TIP

If it's suspected that you are taking in excess air when eating, doctors sometimes recommend watching your swallowing during a meal with a mirror. See whether you are breathing in, rather than out, just before you swallow. If you are, you may need to retrain yourself.

Bloating and Flatulence

Just like burping or belching, bloating and passing gas are normal digestive conditions. Sometimes after eating and definitely when we overeat, we experience feelings of fullness and tightness in the stomach and occasionally feel abdominal pain. This discomfort is usually the result of either swallowed air or stomach and intestinal gas produced by digestion. If the excess air we have swallowed is not released through burping, it may remain in the digestive tract along with any gases present, causing bloat. Because it must be eliminated in some way, it is moved along the alimentary canal through the same peristalsis that moves chyme and feces and is released as *flatus*. The variety of sounds produced during *flatulence* depends on the tightness of the anal sphincter through which the gas is passing and the velocity of the gas as it is expelled.

Sometimes released accidentally while sneezing or coughing, "breaking wind" can certainly be embarrassing and has often been the source of much rude humor.

DEFINITION

Flatus is a mixture of gases expelled from the rectum as a byproduct of the digestive process. **Flatulence** is the expulsion of flatus, or gas.

Getting Down to Gas Roots

Although some people seem to have more gas than others, on average our bodies produce between 1 and 4 pints a day. It's quite normal to expel that gas from 6 to 20 times a day. But where exactly does it all come from, and what accounts for that occasional foul smell? The root of the quantity and quality of the gas we pass is the composition of the food we eat and how our individual bodies break it down.

As previously mentioned, swallowed air accounts for some of the gas, but much of it is a byproduct of your digestion, when broken-down food components mingle with normal bacteria in the colon. In fact, it's the bacteria we can usually blame for the odor, although certain sulfur-containing foods such as eggs, beer, cheese, and cabbage are notorious for producing odorous flatus. Charcoal pills are supposed to absorb smelly sulfurous gas before it is released, and there are even some types of underwear fitted with activated charcoal filters to help alleviate the odor once it arrives. For the most part, however, private expulsion of occasional aromatic flatus is the best bet for eliminating embarrassment.

GI DIDN'T KNOW!

Le Pétomane, also known as the "f'artiste," was a French stage performer of the nineteenth century who had such exceptional control of his flatulence that he was able not only to imitate sounds such as thunder and earthquakes but to "sing" famous tunes as well.

The truth is that many foods, particularly carbohydrates, are gas producing. Cruciferous veggies such as broccoli and cauliflower, whole grains, and fruits such as pears and apples produce gas when digested, and their fiber is usually the cause. Because normal digestion in healthy people relies on a good amount of dietary fiber, we wouldn't want to exclude these foods from our diets. So gas production and the expulsion of it are actually a good thing. Some people, however, cannot properly digest certain foods such as dairy products and experience painful bloating and gas as a result. In these instances, it may be necessary to eliminate the offending foods or substances from their diets (see Chapter 17 on food allergies and intolerance). This type of action may be recommended for those who suffer from celiac or Crohn's disease (CD) as well (see Chapters 8 and 9).

TUMMY TIP

If you are prone to excess gas and bloating after eating beans or other types of healthy carbohydrates, rather than give them up, you may want to take a prescribed or over-the-counter digestive enzyme (Beano is one example) to help prevent your symptoms.

Battling the Bloat

Typical bloating caused by gas, even when occasionally accompanied by sharp abdominal pains, is usually relieved once you are able to burp or pass wind. Sometimes, however, the discomfort is great enough that you may want a little assistance in speeding up the process. Over-the-counter remedies that contain *simethicone*, such as Gas-X, can provide relief by reducing the surface area of gas bubbles and consequently the pressure they exert on the stomach or intestine. Eventually the gas will pass, be absorbed through the intestinal lining, or (if higher up) be relieved with a formidable-sounding belch. Unlike digestive enzymes that can actually reduce the amount of gas, simethicone simply makes it easier to deal with and is for the most part a safe solution for occasional bloating in adults and children alike. Always carefully read the label directions and warnings, however, especially before administering to children as well as adults with other health concerns.

DEFINITION

Simethicone is an antiflatulent present in many over-the-counter antigas medications that can sometimes provide relief from bloating and excess gas. It is normally taken after meals and at bedtime.

It is important, however, to note the difference between a bloated stomach and a distended one. Although a bloated, gaseous tummy can appear distended (stretched and enlarged), not all swollen abdomens are caused by gas. If the distension is continuous rather than intermittent, a specific disease or condition could be at the root of the problem. For example, an organ in the belly area could be enlarged or have a tumor growth, or there could be a collection of fluid in the abdominal region or in the organs themselves. A bowel blockage could also be the cause, resulting in a "plumbing" problem with a buildup of digestive juices and gas. Immediate attention is required for instances such as these, so if you feel that your bloating episodes are more frequent and often unrelated to gas, or if you notice an abdominal enlargement that does not go away, you should see your health practitioner to explore the causes.

Heartburn and Indigestion

Who hasn't reached for the occasional antacid or the fizzy relief of Alka-Seltzer when indigestion—what physicians call dyspepsia—rears its ugly head? Periodic heartburn accompanied by a "sour stomach" or what we often vaguely refer to as "indigestion" is not uncommon. Of the more than 40 percent of Americans who experience this uncomfortable digestive symptom, only about 5 percent actually go to a doctor to treat it. Most of the time, simple over-the-counter remedies offer all the relief we need.

Back Up a Bit

The sensation of heartburn, which is normally felt in the chest just behind the breastbone, is caused by harsh stomach juices coming in contact with the delicate lining of the esophagus. The stomach produces hydrochloric acid in order to digest the food we eat, but occasionally this acid can back up into the throat. There are a number of reasons why this may sometimes occur in the normal course of digestion. Overeating can put pressure on the valve that separates the esophagus from the stomach and cause it to relax and open, allowing stomach fluids to back up. Obesity can put the same type of pressure on the valve, as can lying down or bending over after eating. Some types of food can cause the valve to relax such as chocolate, peppermint, and many spicy and fatty foods. All of these factors can result in stomach acid backwash, or reflux. Thus, the more modern term for heartburn is acid reflux.

GI DIDN'T KNOW!

Sometimes both acid and bile can reflux into the esophagus at the same time when two valves are weak. The pyloric valve separates the small intestine and the stomach, and the lower esophageal valve separates the stomach and the esophagus. Although symptoms are similar and diagnosis may be tricky, bile reflux sometimes causes a gnawing stomach pain that acid reflux does not.

When that fiery feeling of heartburn hits, it's pretty much unmistakable. Often accompanied by a sour taste in the mouth and a bit of burping, we always seem to blame the food we've just eaten and sometimes refer to the experience as "acid indigestion." Whatever you choose to call it and whomever's cooking you wish to blame, infrequent bouts are generally nothing to be concerned about and can usually be quickly dealt with by chewing a few antacids that neutralize acidity and provide immediate relief. Chewing gum may also provide relief through the neutralizing effect of saliva. However, when the experience of heartburn becomes more and more frequent and is accompanied by other symptoms, the possibility of acid reflux disease (see Chapter 5) or the presence of a peptic ulcer (see Chapter 7) may need to be considered by your doctor.

GULP!

Excessive antacid use can have serious consequences. It can alter the effect of other drugs, and calcium-based antacids, when taken in more than the recommended doses, may result in constipation, kidney stones, or (in rare instances) milk-alkali syndrome, a toxic and potentially fatal condition. If you find you are relying heavily on antacids to relieve your heartburn, speak to your doctor right away.

Indigestion or Heart Attack?

At times, the pain you feel with indigestion can be severe. Chest pain, not dissimilar to that felt during a heart attack, may sometimes occur. In these instances, it is critical to proceed as if the pain is a cardiac incident and seek medical attention at once. Tests can easily and immediately differentiate between the two conditions, so it's best to err on the side of caution. If your chest pain turns out to be nothing more than an intense bout of indigestion, a severe gas attack, or even a gallbladder attack, at least you'll be closer to a proper diagnosis so that this type of anxiety-producing pain does not occur again.

TUMMY TIP

Some people who suffer from functional dyspepsia or frequent indigestion find they can avoid symptoms by eliminating fried foods, spicy foods, meats highly marbled with fat, citrus, tomatoes, vinegar, alcohol, and caffeine.

Continual problems with indigestion usually indicate an underlying disease, which can be hard to uncover. Because it encompasses many different types of sensations from heartburn to belching to chest pain, indigestion is often difficult to classify and is often considered to be a functional disorder without an organic, definable cause, once tests have ruled out other conditions. Keeping careful track of your discomfort, including when, where, and how you experience pain, goes a long way to assist your doctor in determining how to address a problem and relieve your symptoms.

Nausea and Vomiting

Nausea is that queasy, uneasy feeling we have all experienced when we announce we are sick to our stomachs and feel as if we may throw up, or vomit, at any moment. Nausea can be one of the most unpleasant sensations we know, often coming on suddenly and causing us to make a beeline to the nearest bathroom. Although nausea and vomiting always seem to spotlight the stomach, in actuality there are a truckload of other reasons why we might feel nausea. Surprisingly, most of these reasons are not even related to digestion.

Don't Rock the Boat

It is true that many digestive conditions cause nausea and vomiting. Stomach virus, irritable bowel syndrome (IBS), celiac disease, liver disease, pancreatitis, colitis, and of course food poisoning are clearly related, as are other digestive causes. Indeed, any condition that irritates the lining of the digestive system can be responsible. But what is interesting about the sensation of nausea—and the possible subsequent vomiting—is the powerful connection between the gut and the brain, a relationship we explored briefly in Chapter 1 and that deserves another look.

For example, motion sickness, which is characterized by severe nausea, dizziness, and often vomiting, has really very little to do with the stomach. The mechanism behind this common phenomenon is that there is a disagreement between what the eyes and the inner ear (which handles equilibrium and balance) perceive. Motion perceived by the eyes does not match that perceived by the ear, and both send contradictory findings to the brain, which decides that somebody must be hallucinating. It makes an executive decision, concluding that the hallucination is due to poison ingestion, and immediately creates an urge, by way of the enteric nervous system, to purge the supposed toxin. It's quite a remarkable response, really.

Other instances in which nausea occurs with no direct connection to digestion are morning sickness (felt by nearly 90 percent of pregnant women, particularly in the first trimester), chemotherapy, drug withdrawal or side effects, stress, depression, and sleep deprivation. Balance disorders that cause dizziness, or *vertigo*, also can result in nausea and vomiting.

DEFINITION

Vertigo is a specific type of dizziness that can result in nausea and vomiting and that is characterized by a sensation of spinning or swaying, even though the body is stationary and motionless.

Purging Complications

The act of purging, or vomiting, can be voluntary or involuntary and is defined as the emptying of the stomach through the esophagus and the mouth. As a consequence, acidic fluids irritate the esophageal lining, just as in acid reflux, and can damage mouth tissue, gums, and tooth enamel if vomiting becomes frequent. People who suffer from eating disorders such as bulimia are particularly at risk for these types of complications. But the greatest danger of continued vomiting, especially if accompanied by diarrhea, is the potential for dehydration. Children are most at risk of becoming dehydrated because, unlike adults, they may not recognize symptoms of dehydration and may fail to replenish themselves with fluids. Sick children should always be checked for visible signs of dehydration such as dry lips, sunken eyes, and decreased or dark urination. In some cases of dehydration in both adults and children, fluid may need to be administered intravenously, including replenishment of *electrolytes*, if moderate to severe symptoms are present.

DEFINITION

Electrolytes (sodium, chloride, potassium, and bicarbonate) are salts normally present in body fluids that are necessary for proper body function. When greatly depleted, organ damage or even death can occur.

Nausea and vomiting that continue for a day or more warrant a doctor's attention. If evidence of red blood or dark blood (that looks like coffee grounds) is present in the vomit, immediate attention is a must. Other accompanying factors—such as running a high fever, abdominal pain, confusion, and respiratory distress—are all signs of a potentially serious condition, so do not waste time in seeking medical help.

TUMMY TIP

Once vomiting has occurred, slowly introduce clear liquids and avoid solid foods until the episode has passed. Get plenty of rest and, with the approval of your doctor, temporarily refrain from taking oral medications that could irritate the stomach and esophagus.

Nipping Nausea in the Bud

When infrequent feelings of simple nausea arise, there are several things you can try yourself before resorting to over-the-counter or prescribed medications. Sipping a sugary, flat drink (such as a soda that has lost its fizz) or munching on plain crackers can often alleviate a mild bout of nausea. Ginger and peppermint have been found to be beneficial in relieving an upset stomach, too (see Chapter 18 on natural remedies). If these are not effective, try purchasing a product such as Pepto-Bismol or Mylanta that coats the stomach lining. For children, purchasing sugar-based remedies such as cola syrup or Emetrol can work quite well. As with all over-the-counter medications, be sure to read and follow label directions carefully. If you are prone to motion sickness, consider taking a mild antinausea medication such as Dramamine just before traveling. This tip may also be useful for nausea that accompanies functional dyspepsia. Stronger, prescribed drugs may be appropriate for other causes of nausea and vomiting, especially if you are being treated with pain medication or chemotherapy for a serious illness.

Constipation and Diarrhea

Although at first it may seem strange to discuss these two seemingly opposite symptoms together, people who often experience constipation also seem to suffer frequent diarrhea. In both instances, the elimination of feces is the issue. Constipation is characterized by infrequent bowel movements that are often hard and painfully passed, usually because of a low intake of fluid and/or fiber in the diet. The longer feces remain in the digestive tract, the more water the colon tends to absorb, adding to the problem. Diarrhea, on the other hand, is characterized by frequent trips to the bathroom that produce loose and watery stools. Temporary bouts of either constipation or diarrhea are actually quite common and are, fortunately, often short lived.

Cause and Effect

According to the American Gastroenterological Association (AGA), as many as 55 million Americans complain of frequent constipation. Why is this so? The same poor eating habits and lack of exercise that have resulted in much of our obesity epidemic are also responsible for many of the common digestive complaints, including constipation. High consumption of processed foods and a diet sorely lacking in fresh fruits, vegetables, and whole grains that can provide healthy dietary fiber are definitely part of the cause. The effect that unhealthy eating has on weight gain and a subsequent inactive lifestyle explains most of the rest.

GULP!

Unexplained weight loss is a symptom that should be reported to your doctor. It could indicate that food is not being properly digested and nutrients are not being absorbed into the bloodstream, typically seen in celiac disease. Other serious diseases could be causing weight loss as well, such as cancer or depression, so always seek medical advice if you are shedding pounds unintentionally.

Surprisingly, the same can be said for diarrhea. Although loose, runny stool can be the result of some forms of medication or an intolerance to foods, particularly dairy, diarrhea is often the result of a virus, parasite, or bacterial infection (see Chapter 15 on food-borne illness). Viruses, bacteria, and toxins are more likely to be picked up when eating out, where both customers and food preparers transfer germs and bacteria through cross contact. If you and your family always eat on the run, resulting in unwanted weight gain and/or occasional constipation and diarrhea, you may want to examine your dining habits. Attempt to improve your diet by eating healthier meals at home more often.

Don't Be Lax

If persistent problems with constipation and diarrhea exist, there could be a more serious underlying condition present. Although it is generally fine to remedy occasional constipation with over-the-counter laxatives, continued use can potentially exacerbate the problem. If you are feeling blocked for more than a week, be sure to see your doctor. Actual blockages in the intestine could be a possibility, or you may need to be evaluated for IBS. The same goes for persistent diarrhea. Periodic use of over-the-counter diarrhea remedies is fine, but you should not rely on them constantly. Most importantly, just as with vomiting, dangerous dehydration as a result of diarrhea can occur after a fairly short time. Be sure to seek medical attention if symptoms last more than 36 to 48 hours. Immediately contact your doctor, however, if you are experiencing bloody (red or black) diarrhea or have an accompanying high fever.

TUMMY TIP

Certain types of drugs such as pain medications (particularly narcotics) are notorious for causing constipation. Your doctor may recommend that you take a stool softener (such as Colace) or a laxative (such as Miralax, which helps push stool forward) to alleviate this side effect.

Abdominal Pain and Cramping

Occasional tummy aches are certainly normal and are typical of constipation and diarrhea. They are usually a sign that we are having trouble digesting something either because we have an intolerance to a food or have consumed too much. A stomach ache could also indicate, however, irritation in the digestive tract. Cramping, generally experienced in the lower GI tract, usually precedes diarrhea and a rush to the bathroom. Painful contractions of the stomach or intestinal muscles can be either acute and sudden or gradual and chronic. For the most part, stomach cramping related to diarrhea disappears once stool is passed. Abdominal pain that is not as transient as cramping and tends to linger, on the other hand, can indicate a wide variety of GI conditions and diseases.

GI DIDN'T KNOW!

Some pains that we experience may not actually be rooted in the area of the body in which we feel the discomfort. This phenomenon is called "referred" or "reflective" pain and is believed to be caused by the sympathetic nervous system. For example, people with a ruptured spleen often feel acute pain in the tip of the left shoulder—an occurrence known as Kehr's sign—while gallbladder pain may be felt in the shoulder, usually the right one, as well.

Point to Where It Hurts

Most of the time, we can zero in on abdominal pain and identify a possible cause by the area of the abdominal cavity where it is felt. For example, pain in the right-upper quadrant may indicate a liver or gallbladder issue. Pain in the left-upper quadrant might suggest something related to the stomach, such as an ulcer, or the spleen, which is also located there. Pain that emanates from the left-lower quadrant could be caused by IBS, diverticulitis, or perhaps a gynecological problem. Pain in the right-lower quadrant may indicate appendicitis or CD. Sometimes, however, you may not be able to pinpoint the area because your pain seems to diffuse over the entire abdominal region. Further probing questions by a health practitioner may assist in preliminary diagnosis and a determination of tests to be conducted. Abdominal pain should never be ignored, and because the causes are many, it's best to start investigating sooner rather than later.

Who You Gonna Call?

Because abdominal pain could require the attention of specialists, seeing your primary physician is normally the best way to proceed—unless, of course, your pain is so severe that an emergency room visit seems warranted. In most cases, however, the primary doctor can do some preliminary testing and refer you to the appropriate physician, whether it be a gastroenterologist, gynecologist, urologist, or someone else who can address your symptoms. Obviously, if you have had any kind of fall or blow to the stomach that brought on your pain, it's important to see someone right away to check for internal organ damage and/or bleeding. Fortunately, most of the time abdominal pain is benign. Emergency rooms report that less than 10 percent of patients who arrive complaining of stomach pain require any serious treatment or surgery. Still, if chronic pain, even in the form of dull aching, is becoming common for you, always get it checked out.

Finding a Gastroenterologist

When symptoms indicate that you need to visit a gastroenterologist, selecting one is not as easy as you may think. You want to receive the best care possible from a physician who has trained at a respectable academic center, has a reputation of excellence, and is board certified. Your primary physician will probably recommend one or two whom he or she knows. Ideally these will be gastroenterologists who got rave reviews from other patients. Family and friends are another source for finding a gastroenterologist, as is the American Gastroenterological Association website (see Appendix B). Do not be reluctant to find the best fit for your needs.

TUMMY TIP

Sometimes the most reliable referrals come from people who actually work on a daily basis with a particular doctor, such as nurses, radiologists, and physician's assistants. Don't be afraid to ask for their unbiased opinions.

Special Attention

A gastroenterologist is an internist who specializes in the diagnosis and treatment of diseases of the digestive system. A gastroenterologist is also trained to perform endoscopic diagnostic and treatment procedures. Board-certified gastroenterologists have not only completed college and medical school, but have trained from three to eight years in gastroenterology at the graduate level and have a good deal of on-the-job hospital training. Licensing exams and certification requirements are rigorous and necessary for accreditation. In the United States, almost all gastroenterologists are board certified in hepatology (the study of the liver, pancreas, and gallbladder) in addition to gastroenterology. A board-certified physician is one who has passed medical board examination after graduation. There are surprisingly many doctors practicing who are not board certified, so be sure to check.

Sometimes gastroenterologists specialize within the field. For example, their expertise may be with celiac and CD or with pediatric gastroenterology. Other specialists who deal with digestive diseases are a hepatologist (for liver disease), a colorectal surgeon (for colon and rectum issues), or an oncologist (for cancer), among others. Most important, however, is how you feel about the special relationship you have with your gastroenterologist or other physician. A trusting and comfortable sense of interaction is essential, especially when dealing with chronic diseases. If you are less than satisfied with your initial meeting, don't hesitate to look elsewhere.

The Bottom Line

Unfortunately, the reality of American health care is that money is the bottom line. If you are lucky enough to have good health insurance, the exorbitant costs of tests and treatment will, for the most part, be covered. But if you have less-than-adequate coverage, state-insured coverage, or no coverage at all, you may encounter difficulties of both a logistical and financial nature that can be terribly discouraging, especially when you are feeling unwell. Know that it is possible, as unpleasant as it is, to challenge the system in order to receive the care you require. Be aware that there are hospitals and clinics, as well as charities, churches, and other philanthropic organizations, that may be able to advocate on your behalf. They can sometimes help you receive the treatment you need as well as some of the funding to pay for it (see Appendix B).

The L

- s that do not necessarily

- e of conditions or diseases

- uld be evaluated by your
  ogist or other specialist.

- medical attention or a visit

- t fit for you. Get recom-
  edge.

- ir evaluations. Seek help if
  e.

Welcome to Thompson Public
Library
www.thompsonpubliclibrary.org
860.923.9779

A receipt of your transaction:

You checked out the following
items:

1. The complete idiot's guide to
   digestive health
   Call No.:
   Barcode: 34038118792308
   Due: 5/14/2021
2. Crohn's and colitis for
   dummies
   Call No.:
   Barcode: 34038118600857
   Due: 5/14/2021

TOMPSN 4/23/2021 3:33 PM

Visiting the Gastroenterologist

In This Chapter

- Preparing for your first appointment
- Common tests your gastroenterologist will likely perform
- Other possible diagnostic tests you may encounter

Once you determine that a visit to the gastroenterologist is in order and you select the one to see, you probably want to know what's likely to happen next and how to be a proactive participant in your own health care. A basic understanding of gastroenterological procedures and jargon goes a long way in improving your interaction with the gastroenterologist, enabling you to ask probing and thoughtful questions during your initial and subsequent visits.

In this chapter, you'll learn what your first visit will be like and will explore various types of tests your gastroenterologist may prescribe and why. We'll also look at what your results might indicate and how they could relate to symptoms you have. From blood work and imaging to the dreaded colonoscopy, you'll be well versed in the technological diagnostics you may encounter as you work with your gastroenterologist to discover the cause of your distress and begin to treat your conditions or illness.

We are fortunate to live in a time when modern medicine is advancing in leaps and bounds nearly every day. As a result, conditions that were once misunderstood or labeled untreatable can now be cured and even prevented. Similarly, many surgical techniques that were once complicated and dangerous, requiring much recuperative time and therapy, have been replaced with modern techniques that sometimes require only a day's stay in the hospital. We have more reason than ever to be hopeful that our health problems can be addressed and remedied.

Preparation Is Everything

A good physician appreciates your input, so it's of utmost importance to be prepared for your initial visit. Prepare not only paperwork and documentation but also a well-thought-out verbal description of what you feel and experience. The more you are able to share about your condition and specific physical issues, the better your gastroenterologist will be able to analyze your problem. In particular, don't be afraid to share embarrassing symptoms that seem private, such as bathroom habits, for these are often critical signs of certain conditions or diseases. As you tell your story, the gastroenterologist will no doubt ask specific questions in order to explore something significant, so don't hold anything back. Be honest and accurate and never hide any pain or discomfort that is real to you, even though you may fear it makes you look weak. Everyone has different thresholds of pain and different tolerance levels. If something is bothering you, as small as it may seem, it is definitely worth mentioning.

TUMMY TIP

So you don't forget any details you want to share, begin jotting down your thoughts as they come to you a week or more before your visit or keep a small tape recorder handy to speak into and transcribe from later.

The Paper Trail

Despite the digital nature of our world in nearly every other area, medical documentation on paper is still the norm. Plan to bring the following papers with you:

- Your most up-to-date insurance card
- A referral form from your primary doctor, if required
- Copies of recent blood work
- Other test results such as x-rays
- A list of medications you are taking
- A food or symptom diary or journal

In addition, you may need to bring a photo ID, past medical records, dates of previous surgeries or hospital stays, and notes about any medications you are allergic to or with which you have had unacceptable side effects.

GI DIDN'T KNOW!

Medical records from other doctors' offices are the property of those offices and can only be transferred with your authorization. Consequently, you must sign a release form (either at the new or old doctor's office) in order to have any files transferred.

You'll no doubt be asked to fill out an extensive questionnaire about your medical history when you arrive at the gastroenterologist's office. Many of the documents listed previously will help you to complete the forms. This rather tedious trail of paper is unfortunately necessary, but the good news is that future visits will be virtually paper free.

Readying Yourself

Now that your paperwork is in order, it's time to prepare yourself. When you make your appointment, you will learn whether you should eat or drink prior to your visit. Fasting (not eating or perhaps even drinking) is necessary for certain tests. Be sure to adhere strictly to any of these instructions. You may be asked to bring a stool sample, and in some cases, lab work may be requested before you even arrive. In most cases, however, your gastroenterologist will want to meet with you first and give you a general exam before deciding on which, if any tests, to conduct.

You may want to consider bringing a friend or family member, particularly if you have a difficult time remembering things. At the very least, bring a notepad and pen so you can write down anything you want to be sure to recall. It may also be helpful to bring along your personal calendar if any tests are planned, so you can check your schedule for availability. Finally, be sure to bring an open mind to the experience. It will be your most important asset as you interact with your doctor and work together with him to resolve your digestive problem.

The General Examination

As is the case with many doctor visits, you can expect to have your height and weight measured and your blood pressure taken, and you will be asked to disrobe partially in preparation for the doctor. A good doctor will have already looked at your paperwork before entering the room and have a general idea as to why you are there, but he or she will probably still want to hear the nature of the problem directly from you. Try to be as specific as possible when discussing pain and be sure to include other feelings you may be experiencing such as fatigue or depression. These feelings could provide clues that help the gastroenterologist to make a preliminary diagnosis.

Palpable Probing

Depending on what symptoms you report, the gastroenterologist may listen to your lungs, heart, and abdomen with a stethoscope. He or she will then start doing a little palpable probing, feeling and pressing around your upper and lower abdomen, looking for anything significant and obvious such as lumps or fluid buildup. You may or may not feel pain or discomfort, but if you do, be sure to say so and to what degree. Use specific words like "sharp" or "burning" as opposed to simply "it hurts." Any tenderness you feel during a palpable exam may or may not resemble the actual discomfort you came to discuss. Sometimes until firm pressure is applied in certain areas of the body, we don't realize there is any tenderness. Be sure to note if this is the case or if the pain is indeed the same as that you've been having.

GI DIDN'T KNOW!

Doctors listen to your belly with a stethoscope to detect irregularities as well as normal sounds of stomach grumbling called borborygmi. This odd term is named for the sounds caused by muscle contractions in the digestive tract during its "housecleaning" phase between meals.

In some cases, you will have a digital rectal examination (DRE) at your first visit. Although a bit uncomfortable, a DRE is usually quick and painless. Using a gloved and lubricated finger, the gastroenterologist probes the inside of the rectum, feeling for tumors or other abnormalities. The outside of the rectum (anus) may also be checked for hemorrhoids or rashes. If you are undergoing a colonoscopy in the near future, however, your gastroenterologist may choose to skip the DRE at this time.

Assessing the Situation

In some instances, the gastroenterologist may have all the information he or she needs to make a proper assessment about the causes of your distress. Conditions such as mild acid reflux disease may simply require a prescribed medicine, diet recommendations, and a return visit. In other cases, the initial visit may be just the beginning of getting to the root of your problem. Other diagnostic tests may be necessary. Other than having blood drawn, it's unlikely you will undergo any further testing at this time. If you need more tests, the gastroenterologist usually writes a prescription for specific tests needed, and the office will probably be able to help you make arrangements for them. Most doctors have diagnostic centers or hospitals that they normally use and trust. Depending on the test, it may be possible to schedule something quite soon, or in some instances, there may be a waiting period. Preparation may also be necessary, as in the case of a colonoscopy, and you will receive important details from the office before you go.

If it is not clear to you, ask why the doctor has ordered certain tests and what he or she is looking to find. Often a proper diagnosis requires eliminating other possibilities, and it may be the case that some tests, both *invasive* and *noninvasive*, are ordered for this reason. Finding an immediate answer to your problem is often not possible, so try to be a "patient" patient and at least be glad that the process is finally underway.

DEFINITION

Medically speaking, **noninvasive** tests are those that do not penetrate the body cavity in a significant way, such as breath, blood, and imaging tests like x-rays and scans. **Invasive** tests include procedures such as endoscopic probes, including colonoscopy, and tests such as biopsies in which tissue is collected for examination.

It's in the Blood

A lot can be learned about your health from your body's blood, from fighting an infection to a lower-than-normal presence of certain vitamins and minerals. For the gastroenterologist, blood work can further assist an initial assessment by revealing particular abnormalities that are either significant on their own or that indicate poor digestion. If you have ever seen a lab report of your blood work requested by your family doctor or specialist, you know that it is next to impossible for the average Joe to decipher. Because we don't normally have a clue as to what we're looking at, except for maybe our cholesterol numbers, we tend to focus on the parts that say "low" or "high," indicating we are out of normal range. Rather than gasping with concern, it's best to leave the interpretation to professionals who evaluate any abnormal findings and determine if they require further investigation. Still, it's not a bad idea to ask for a copy for your files in case other physicians you end up seeing request a recent lab test.

Common Indicators

The most common type of blood test requested by a doctor is a complete blood count (CBC). This test provides information about the cells in your blood, specifically white blood cells, red blood cells, and platelets. Fluctuations in these counts can indicate the presence of a number of diseases, but your gastroenterologist will be particularly interested in checking for *anemia*. Anemia could indicate blood loss from the digestive tract. Your doctor would also be interested in noting whether your white blood cell count is elevated, which could indicate the presence of infection or inflammation. Similarly, a low platelet count could indicate serious liver disease.

DEFINITION

Anemia is the general term that refers to a decrease in red blood cells caused by any of several reasons and characterized by a general feeling of weakness and fatigue.

Another common blood test is the comprehensive metabolic panel (CMP). The CMP is a broad screening that includes 14 specific blood tests. Fasting is normally required before blood is drawn for this test. Indicators such as serum glucose, calcium, and blood urea nitrogen, to name a few, can shed light on the health of your liver and kidneys and give a good idea of your nutritional state. For example, chronic diarrhea could result in low potassium levels. Any abnormalities in this test need to be evaluated within the context of your digestive problems and may help to determine initial treatment and/or further diagnostic tests to conduct.

Other Blood Relations

Although there are numerous other specific blood tests that might reveal a relationship to your symptoms, the following are those that your gastroenterologist may find particularly helpful in assessing your condition:

- C-reactive protein (CRP) is an additional marker of inflammation and infection and is produced by the liver.

- Elevated lipase enzymes could indicate problems with the pancreas or gastroenteritis.

- Immunoglobulin A (IgA) and antitransglutaminase antibodies (ATA) are strong indicators of celiac disease.

- Low vitamin B$_{12}$ levels could suggest Crohn's disease (CD) or pernicious anemia.

- Low vitamin D levels are sometimes associated with chronic pain, particularly in women.

In addition, testing the thyroid gland can be helpful in determining the cause of some bowel dysfunctions. An underactive thyroid (hypothyroidism) can be responsible for constipation, while an overactive thyroid (hyperthyroidism) could result in bouts of diarrhea. Finally, the presence of *H. pylori* antibodies in the blood indicates exposure to these bacteria, which are now accepted as the primary cause of numerous upper gastrointestinal (GI) disorders, including peptic ulcers, gastritis, and even stomach cancer (see Chapter 7).

GI DIDN'T KNOW!

Dr. Barry Marshall of Australia and his pathologist, Robin Warren, won the 2005 Nobel Prize in medicine for discovering that *H. pylori* was the actual cause of most gastritis and ulcers, not stress or food as previously believed. To convince the medical community, Dr. Marshall drank a beaker of *H. pylori* and became seriously ill. Subsequent self-testing revealed he was correct.

Take the Breath Test

Noninvasive breath tests can often shed light on a few specific symptoms you may experience, although these breath tests tend to be used less frequently in modern gastroenterology. They are typically safe for everyone, including children and pregnant women, and may be ordered by your gastroenterologist to detect conditions such as lactose intolerance and *H. pylori*. Normally, a fasting period of 8 to 12 hours before the test is necessary, and certain medications should not be taken during that time. In addition, taking antibiotics a few weeks prior to the test may reduce its accuracy.

Hydrogen Exhalation

One type of breath test involves the detection of hydrogen gas. Under normal circumstances, people do not exhale hydrogen, but when there exists an intolerance to lactose or fructose, hydrogen is produced as a byproduct in the colon. It is then absorbed from the digestive tract into the bloodstream and finally into the lungs, where it is released during exhalation. This test involves drinking a lactose-loaded beverage, after which your breath is analyzed at intervals for the presence of hydrogen.

> **GULP!**
>
> Hydrogen breath tests for lactose and fructose are apt to cause side effects, as would be expected in patients who suffer from these types of intolerance. These effects include bloating, pain, and diarrhea. Lactulose tests, however, cause few side effects as the dose administered is quite small.

Another hydrogen breath test, sometimes referred to as a lactulose test, is occasionally done when there is a suspicion of small intestinal bacterial overgrowth (SIBO). In this circumstance, bacteria in the small intestine compete with you for your nutrients. The idea is that, normally, the small intestine is sterile and there should be no bacteria there to compete with you to absorb the nutrients you are digesting. A positive lactulose breath test may indicate a rapid transit of food to colon from stomach. The idea of the breath tests is that if your body digests the sugars, then you don't breathe out the hydrogen. If you can't digest the sugars, the bacteria in your colon do their own type of digestion that produces hydrogen, which can be detected in exhaled air. How the test works is that it measures the time from ingestion of lactulose until the time you breathe it out. If the test detects the hydrogen early on, it either means that there are bacteria in the small intestine that are digesting and absorbing the nutrients (i.e., lactulose), or that the ingested food is going more quickly than normal from stomach to colon. This rapid transit can be a feature of irritable bowel syndrome (IBS).

When you take these tests, you breathe into a bag that is then sealed, providing a baseline level of the gas to be measured. Then you consume the sugar in question—or urea in case of *H. pylori*—and then after a certain amount of time (or several times, ranging from 15 minutes to hours), you breathe back into the bag. Your doctor can compare your baseline to these levels to detect a problem. They are noninvasive tests, but they can take a while. However, the relevance of SIBO has recently come into question as a primary cause of IBS, so some gastroenterologists may take the results of this test, if they decide to conduct it at all, with a grain of salt in their assessment of your condition.

The Urea Breath Test

The urea breath test shows the presence of *H. pylori* bacteria. It is more telling than a blood test because a positive outcome indicates the bacteria are actually present in your system. The blood test, which looks for antibodies, can reveal that you were exposed to *H. pylori* at some point in your life, but may not reveal if they are still present. This is why the urea breath test is one of the best ways to discover if the bacteria have been eradicated after antibiotic treatment, which a blood test might not prove. Highly sensitive and accurate, the test can be tremendously helpful in diagnosing and treating gastritis as well as gastric and peptic ulcers.

Examining Stool

Your fecal matter can shed light on a number of digestive symptoms. Stool examination can reveal the presence of parasites or bacteria and can provide clues to lactose intolerance and colorectal or stomach cancer, among other conditions. The collection of fecal matter is sometimes done at the doctor's office or at a medical facility. Home diagnostic tests are also available from your physician, hospitals, and even over-the-counter in some drugstores. Often a special diet is required up to two days before the test. For some types of tests, you may be asked to collect stool samples over a period of hours or days.

Occult Happenings

A fecal occult blood test (FOBT) checks for hidden, or occult, blood in the stool, which can indicate a subtle loss of blood in the digestive tract. This very sensitive test picks up blood presence not normally seen by the naked eye. A positive result requires further checking for polyps or ulcers and can often be a sign of cancer of the colon or rectum. Unfortunately, both false positives and false negatives can occur with the FOBT if a patient doesn't follow strict dietary restrictions prior to the test. For example, the ingestion of red meat can alter results, as can eating certain vegetables and fruits such as cabbage, horseradish, or cantaloupe. Similarly, vitamin C supplements and citrus may produce a falsely negative result. Still, as a noninvasive test, the FOBT is generally performed before other invasive tests.

A Cultural Phenomenon

Certain types of fecal tests called stool cultures can be helpful in determining the cause of symptoms such as bloody diarrhea, nausea, vomiting, and abdominal pain. These cultures can reveal the presence of bacteria such as those associated with food poisoning like the *E. coli* strain 0157:H7, or they can show the presence of parasites. Sometimes a person can be a symptom-free carrier of bacteria and not seem infected. A culture can indicate this condition as well and is an important test for people in the food industry who could potentially infect others.

Another stool test called a pH test can point to lactose intolerance, particularly in infants and children, when acid levels are particularly high. In addition, a fecal fat test can indicate whether fats are absorbed properly by the digestive system; if not, the result could be unexplained weight loss, belly distention, scaly skin, and *steatorrhea*. This condition could be caused by a problem with the pancreas or the small intestine, such as sprue or CD, and would prompt further testing.

DEFINITION

Steatorrhea is the presence of excess fat in stool, which causes feces to float, appear oily, and be especially foul smelling. Anal leakage may also occur. Fat substitutes in commercial foods as well as some diet medications can result in steatorrhea.

X-Rays and Imaging

As a follow-up or in conjunction with simple blood work, breath exams, or stool tests, it may be necessary to get a closer look inside your body. Your gastroenterologist may order x-rays and/or other radiological tests such as computed tomography (CT) scans, as well as ultrasound or magnetic resonance imaging (MRI). In addition to assisting in a proper diagnosis, imaging tests are useful in the management of disease once it is pinpointed and are often used during certain types of surgeries and procedures.

Although much of modern medicine has turned its focus toward high-quality imaging, simple x-rays are still valuable tools in discovering causes of digestive discomfort, particularly in emergency situations. A quick abdominal x-ray can rule out the presence of air in the abdominal cavity, which could indicate something like a ruptured bowel. An x-ray can also reveal a blockage in the intestine and occasionally even show kidney stones or gallstones when they are prominent.

Barium Cocktail

Some of the oldest types of GI tests that involve imaging are the barium swallow or barium enema, also known as an upper or lower GI series. Depending on which portion of the digestive tract your doctor wishes to examine, you either drink a contrast medium or receive an enema containing barium sulfate. This substance appears white during imaging and contrasts with the gray areas of organs and black areas of air.

As the solution travels through your digestive system, the doctor or *radiologist* views the process in real time using a fluoroscope connected to a monitor. This process allows the observation of any abnormalities in flow from the esophagus to the upper small intestine or from the colon to the lower small intestine. Periodic x-rays are taken as well. Tumors, polyps, and blockages associated with CD are often found using this method. The drawback, however, is that any growths discovered cannot be biopsied or removed during the test, which could be done if viewed during a colonoscopy. Unfortunately, some insurance providers insist on a GI series before approving the more costly scope procedures.

DEFINITION

A **radiologist** is a medical doctor who specializes in the reading and interpretation of x-rays and other types of imaging. Radiologists are usually specialists in a particular area such as mammography, cardiac imaging, or GI imaging.

The CAT's Meow

Since the 1970s, a remarkable imaging technique known as computed axial tomography (CAT)—or simply computed tomography (CT)—has allowed unique views of the human body. While you are lying down, a rotating x-ray device creates cross-sectional images of bones, organs, or other body parts that your doctor wants to view in greater detail. Like thin slices taken from a large salami, each image can be neatly separated from the whole, displayed, and examined for abnormalities. Gastroenterologists often use CT scans to look for tumors or inflammation, and scabs are particularly helpful in detecting pancreatic cancer and enlarged lymph nodes. The unfortunate downside of this type of imaging is the enormous amount of radiation to which the patient is exposed. A single scan is roughly equivalent to 300 chest x-rays. When necessary, however, CT scans are invaluable as incredibly accurate diagnostic tools and are excellent for monitoring the progression of diseases.

GULP!

A recent study suggests that the amount of radiation generated from multiple CT scans is equivalent to the exposure that survivors in Nagasaki and Hiroshima received from the atomic bomb. If you are concerned about radiation exposure, be sure to speak with your doctor about the pros and cons of this type of testing.

3D Imaging

Magnetic resonance imaging (MRI) is another testing procedure that allows for cross-sectional or three-dimensional views of the body. Unlike CT scans, MRI does not expose the patient to radiation. Rather, it works through powerful magnetic fields to create contrast between the compositions of soft tissue. Although fine detail is limited, this imaging technique lends itself quite well to investigating disorders of the liver, pancreas, spleen, gallbladder, and biliary tract. When these areas are the focus, the test is referred to as—get ready for this—magnetic resonance cholangiopancre-atography (yikes!). Called MRCP for short (phew!), this test is particularly good for looking at ducts and finding tumors that may be cancerous.

Another type of MRI used in the field of gastroenterology is the abdominal MR angiogram. This test is great for discerning blood flow problems in the gut and evaluating any *aortic aneurysms* that may be present. Often there are no symptoms with this type of aneurysm, although occasionally back or stomach pain may be present. Serious rupture resulting in hemorrhage and quick death can occur if not treated, so this test can often be a real life saver. And, unlike coronary angiograms that are used to evaluate heart disease, the abdominal MR angiogram is quite safe and fast as well as much less expensive.

DEFINITION

An **aortic aneurysm** is a swelling or dilation of an area in the main artery of the body, which indicates a weakness in the artery wall.

The Sound of Waves

Ultrasound testing is used in a variety of medical situations, most familiarly in obstetrics when a mom-to-be gets her first look at the baby growing within her. Ultrasound works by sending high-frequency sound waves that reflect off the body, creating a black and white picture. Ultrasound testing is useful in certain GI situations as well. Sometimes called abdominal sonography, this type of test is excellent at detecting gallstones and imaging the liver, gallbladder, spleen, pancreas, and kidneys. Usually performed by technicians called sonographers, ultrasound tests are conducted while the patient is lying down. A gel that conducts the sound waves goes on the abdomen while a handheld transducer or probe scans the internal organs from the outside, images of which appear on a nearby monitor.

GI DIDN'T KNOW!

High-frequency sound waves produced by ultrasound testing can be heard by some animals, including dogs, cats, dolphins, bats, and mice.

Esophagogastroduodenoscopy, Huh?

This impossible-to-pronounce test is (thank goodness!) also referred to as an upper GI endoscopy, or EGD. It allows the doctor to make a thorough examination of your esophagus, stomach, and duodenum (the upper part of your small intestine). Endoscopies in general have drastically changed the face of modern medicine and are indispensable tools in the early detection of serious diseases, including cancer. They are considered to be minimally invasive procedures that allow a close-up look at the interior surface of organs and are performed via insertion of a long, flexible tube into a body cavity. The tube has a light on its end connected to a camera chip that transmits an image to a TV screen. In the case of an upper GI endoscopy, your doctor may order this test if, for example, you have acid reflux symptoms that can't seem to be managed very well with medication, especially if you are over the age of 50.

GI DIDN'T KNOW!

Stomach cancer is so prevalent in Japan that many people schedule a routine upper GI endoscopy, often during their lunch breaks. Consequently, most patients abstain from sedation so they can get right back to work.

Scoping Things Out

The EGD is a great diagnostic tool for detecting the cause of upper GI bleeding, persistent dyspepsia, difficulty or pain in swallowing, and chronic acid reflux. It is the best way to check for cell abnormalities associated with Barrett's esophagus (see Chapter 6). It can also be helpful in monitoring the progress of upper GI conditions or diseases and may even be used therapeutically to stop bleeding or to remove a foreign object in the upper portion of the digestive tract. The flexible tube can move around quite well and catch a view of just about anything it happens to meet along its path. The EGD is often valuable in eliminating the possibility of conditions that mimic symptoms you may be experiencing, helping your doctor get a quicker and better diagnosis.

Numb Me Up

Before the endoscope is inserted into your mouth and down the esophagus, the back of the throat is numbed with a local anesthetic to prevent gagging. You'll also be moderately sedated and relatively unaware of the entire procedure. Fasting before the EGD is required—usually at least four to six hours to give the stomach a chance to empty and prevent aspiration of food down the windpipe. Your heart rate, blood pressure, and oxygen levels are monitored. You may also receive oxygen through a tube in your nose.

The procedure itself lasts about 30 minutes. After a brief stay in the recovery room, you'll be on your way home with little more than a mild sore throat and a few yawns. Still, it's best to have someone available to drive you home. During the EGD, your doctor may remove questionable tissue for further testing, referred to as a biopsy. Once a pathologist has had a chance to process the tissue and examine it under a microscope, you'll be informed of the biopsy results, but your gastroenterologist may inform you of the general results of the EGD once you are awake.

The Dreaded Colonoscopy

More dreadful things have been said about colonoscopies than we can shake a probe at, but frankly, these diagnostic tests (and often therapeutic tests), as uncomfortable as they may be, save lives that years ago would have been lost to cancer. Studies have shown that a colonoscopy reveals polyps (potentially precancerous growths) that a barium test cannot, making colonoscopies instrumental in early detection. Like the EGD, a colonoscopy is an endoscopic procedure except that the tube used is thicker and longer and is inserted into the anus and not the mouth. The preparation required for a colonoscopy is more extensive and considerably more unpleasant, which is the primary reason it has received such a bad rap.

Here, Drink This

For your doctor to get a good view of your colon, as well as the lower small intestine and rectum, it's necessary for the passageway to be pristinely clean, and this is where the unpleasantness comes. The only way to clear out all fecal matter is by inducing diarrhea. An oral laxative is the norm, also called a lavage or bowel prep solution, although enemas are also possible. Prior to the laxative you'll consume a clear liquid diet for at least one day and eliminate high-fiber foods, such as corn, from your meals a day or two before that. You will get detailed instructions and information from the doctor's office as to when you should begin and discontinue certain medications. Don't hesitate, however, to ask for clarification if any of the instructions are confusing. The last thing you want is to have to redo the preparation because it was done incorrectly the first time.

The day before your procedure, plan to park yourself near a bathroom as you'll spend most of your time there. Using medicated wipes rather than toilet tissue can ease some of the irritation you may feel from continual wiping. Keep yourself hydrated with clear liquids only—colors and flavorings could alter the test results. Enough can't be said about following the directions you have been given, so get them as early as you can and read them as carefully as you can—more than two or three times if necessary.

Up We Go

The day of your procedure you still need to refrain from food, but you may be able to drink something until four to six hours before the test. As with the EGD, you receive a moderate sedative to relax you, and you lie on your left side. The tube, or colonoscope, all 5 feet of it, is inserted slowly and guided into the colon. The only discomfort you may feel is a little bit of gas or a tugging sensation. You may also feel an urge to defecate, but don't worry—there's nothing there to expel. Occasionally you may be asked to change your position ever so slightly, but for the most part you'll get through the 20- to 30-minute procedure without any real awareness of what is happening. This state is called conscious or procedural sedation, and it is used in other medical procedures as well that would be unpleasant if one were wide awake. Most doctors use propofol for sedation, and patients usually have no awareness or recollection.

If your doctor finds any polyps in your colon, the goal is to remove them during the procedure unless they are worrisome or very large. Polyps are removed by either a biopsy or a snare, a metal lasso-type instrument that uses electricity to help cut and coagulate tissue at the same time.

End Results

Although the main purpose of a colonoscopy is to check for the presence of polyps, there are other conditions that your gastroenterologist may wish to investigate. Suspicion of inflammatory bowel disease, signs of anemia, or unexplained changes in your bowel habits could also prompt a colonoscopy. Under some circumstances, your gastroenterologist may wish to collect tissue from the lining of the colon or any other part of the lower GI tract. Any samples taken will be processed by a pathologist, and the results, as with EGD biopsies, will be available in a few days. Otherwise, your doctor can report the general results to you almost immediately once you are in the recovery room. The sedation requires that someone drive you home, and you may feel a bit bloated for a while, but otherwise you'll bounce back quite quickly. Refrain from drinking alcohol, however, for the remainder of the day and avoid any critical physical or mental activities as well, such as heavy lifting or signing contracts.

GULP!

Serious complications from colonoscopies, such as perforations or holes in the colon, are extremely rare. More common, although still relatively rare, is the possibility of bleeding after polyp or tissue removal. If you experience rectal bleeding, fever or chills, or severe abdominal pain, contact your doctor immediately.

Other Procedures and Tests

Although we've covered the major GI tests and then some, there are certainly many, many more that are possible depending on your symptoms and what the doctor suspects could be causing them. The following are a few more diagnostic tools available to your gastroenterologist that you may or may not encounter.

Sigmoidoscopy

This procedure is like an abbreviated colonoscopy and can actually be done in the doctor's office. A short, flexible tube with a camera is inserted through the anus and into the sigmoid portion of the colon (the lower 24 inches or so). Sometimes used as a screening tool before the recommendation of a colonoscopy, this test can detect polyps, inflammation, and other abnormalities. No sedation is required, but the lower colon area must be cleared with an enema. Often quite uncomfortable, sigmoidoscopies are performed less and less since colonoscopies have become common.

Manometry

When the proper functioning of a sphincter, or valve, is in question, either in the esophagus or colon, this test may be ordered. It is also ideal for detecting motility problems, as it measures the pressure of contractions that take place in these areas.

For esophageal manometry, a catheter is inserted into the stomach through the nose which is then slowly withdrawn, noting changes in pressure. For colonic manometry, often called amorectal manometry, a tube is placed in the colon through the rectum. A balloon is inserted into the anus and filled until the patient can feel it, and the volume is recorded. The tube is filled more until the patient says it hurts, and the volume is recorded. Finally, a patient expels the balloon. Manometry tests may indicate the presence of certain conditions such as spasms, incontinence, visceral hypersensitivity, *achalasia*, or abnormalities of the pelvic floor. Fasting is normally required prior to manometry, as well as an enema if the colon is being examined.

DEFINITION

Achalasia is a disorder of the esophagus characterized by difficulty swallowing, an inability to belch, or regurgitation that gets progressively worse, resulting in weight loss, coughing when lying down, and chest pain.

HIDA Scan

Technically called a cholescintigraphy scan, a HIDA is a nuclear study of the bile ducts that checks for obstruction by gallstones, scar tissue, or tumors or detects bile leaks after a gallbladder has been removed. It is also used to detect chronic gallbladder problems when other tests are normal. A radioactive agent, referred to as a bile tracer, is injected intravenously and then followed with a camera placed over the abdomen as it works its way into ducts and organs, including the liver. If the tracer fails to enter certain areas, obstruction is probable.

Candid Camera

One of the more interesting tests developed in recent years is the small bowel capsule endoscopy, or capsule camera. It presents a whole new way to view the inside of the digestive tract and even reveals areas that are not visible by other endoscopic procedures. Essentially, you swallow a pill that has a video camera and light source in it. As it makes its incredible journey, a wireless connection allows it to send back images to a gizmo you wear on your waist. After eight hours or so when the battery wears out, your doctor connects the collected images to a computer and downloads them for his viewing pleasure. Eventually the pill is eliminated and down the drain it goes. The result: your very own digestive documentary.

GULP!

Because the capsule camera is able to detect the smallest evidence of gastro-intestinal bleeding, one of the most important findings since its use began is the extent to which nonsteroidal anti-inflammatory drugs (NSAIDs) such as ibu-profen can damage the small bowel—much greater, in fact, than once believed.

The Least You Need to Know

- Preparation for your initial visit with the gastroenterologist is an important factor in getting a satisfactory result.
- Simple tests that examine your blood, breath, and stool may reveal quite a bit about your digestive problems.
- Depending on your symptoms, the gastroenterologist may order further testing to reach a conclusive diagnosis.
- From imaging tests to endoscopies, there is no shortage of diagnostic tools available to the modern gastroenterologist.

Upper GI Conditions and Diseases

Now that you're acquainted with your body's digestive system, it's time to take a closer look at some conditions and diseases that you or someone you know may have. Here we'll focus on the upper gastrointestinal area of the digestive system, namely the esophagus, stomach, and upper small intestine, where conditions such as acid reflux disease and gastritis occur. You'll learn about typical symptoms as well as how your doctor will most likely diagnose and treat what he or she finds.

We'll also cover a few quite serious digestive diseases, such as Barrett's esophagus and stomach cancer, as well as celiac disease. We'll talk about diagnosis, treatment, and reducing your risk factors in the first place. Current studies and the latest effective treatments and medications will be discussed, too. With the information you have in hand, you'll definitely be well versed in the facts.

Acid Reflux Disease

In This Chapter

- Knowing when your heartburn warrants worry
- Getting medical treatment for acid reflux disease
- Making changes for relief and prevention

When the hassle of heartburn becomes more than occasional and over-the-counter remedies prove less and less effective, you may be a candidate for a diagnosis of acid reflux disease. Also known as gastroesophageal reflux disease (GERD), acid reflux disease is a more serious condition that's worth your worry. Acidic stomach contents back up (reflux) into the esophagus, causing irritation and frequent heartburn. If it's any consolation, you are definitely not alone. According to the National Institutes of Health, nearly 60 million Americans experience symptoms of acid reflux disease, or simply reflux disease, at least once a month.

Whatever you've heard about GERD, it's definitely on the rise. As we continue to grow as a nation—weight-wise, that is—so does the frequency of many digestive disorders, including GERD. Although obesity is a definite risk factor, there is much more to this potentially dangerous disease than meets the eye. In this chapter, we'll take a good look at GERD: what it is, how it's detected and treated, and what you can do right now to help prevent it from becoming your diagnosis.

Acid on the Rise

As with most common complaints of heartburn, acid lies at the root of a GERD sufferer's problem. Stomach acid, somewhere between the potency of lemon juice and battery acid, rises into the esophagus, irritating its delicate lining. Although the formidably tough interior wall of the stomach is designed to handle this acidity, your esophagus cannot. As a result, after a period of continued irritation, the esophageal lining becomes inflamed and ultimately damaged. If left untreated, complications such as ulcers, bleeding, *dysphagia*, and possibly esophageal cancer can result.

DEFINITION

Dysphagia is the medical term for difficulty swallowing.

Blame It on the Sphincter

What causes the acid in your stomach to back up into the esophagus? More often than not, acid reflux occurs because of a problem with the lower esophageal sphincter (LES). This valve, located at the bottom of your esophagus, is a kind of sentry that is supposed to open the door only to allow food and liquids to enter the stomach when you swallow (and permit the occasional belch back out) and then close the door to keep any stomach acid from escaping. Unfortunately, sometimes the sphincter is either weak or lazy, and those powerful acidic stomach fluids get past it into the esophagus. Usually, the severity of your acid reflux depends on how well the sphincter is doing its job. Certain types of medications, fatty foods, coffee, smoking, and alcohol abuse are just a few things that can relax and weaken the LES's performance.

Other factors besides a faulty sphincter can cause acid backup, too. The neutralizing effect of your saliva may not be effective enough, or the amount of stomach acid produced during digestion may prove overwhelming, such as in the rare condition known as *Zollinger-Ellison syndrome*. Obesity and pregnancy can also be factors. Pressure from excess weight can cause stomach acid to escape into the esophagus and may affect the proper functioning of other digestive organs as well. In most cases, however, we can blame it on the esophageal sphincter.

DEFINITION

Zollinger-Ellison syndrome is a rare disorder in which a tumor releases a hormone that leads to extraordinary amounts of stomach acid, often resulting in severe acid reflux. It is named after two Ohio State University surgeons, Robert Zollinger and Edwin Ellison, who first described the condition in 1955.

Symptoms to Watch For

Although frequent heartburn (several times a week) is by far the most common symptom of GERD, here are some other warning signs:

- Unexplained chest pain, particularly at night
- Difficulty swallowing (dysphagia)
- Excessive belching
- Persistent cough or hoarseness
- Wheezing or asthma-type symptoms
- Sour taste or food regurgitation

The following symptoms require immediate medical attention:

- Severe dysphagia
- Vomiting of blood
- Black stool
- Weight loss

Although many of the preceding symptoms can be a result of other unrelated conditions, when accompanied by severe and chronic heartburn, there is a good chance they may be connected.

GI DIDN'T KNOW!

GERD is not just an adult's disease. Children, including infants, can also develop GERD, although in some cases it can be tricky to diagnose. Spitting up, sore throat, and food avoidance are a few of the signs.

Diagnosing GERD

Explaining your symptoms to the doctor, as well as reporting your limited success or failure with over-the-counter remedies for relief, is usually enough for the diagnosis of GERD. You will probably get a prescription medicine—most likely an acid suppressant—to take for at least a few weeks and sometimes up to 12 weeks, and you will be advised on lifestyle changes you can make. However, if your doctor feels that your symptoms are severe enough, or if the prescribed medications are ultimately of little help, further testing may be necessary.

Possible tests that your gastroenterologist may conduct include an upper endoscopy (EGD), a pH test called a Bravo probe, or a barium x-ray. The endoscopy, usually the first line of inquiry, can indicate the extent of tissue damage and, in fact, for patients over the age of 50 experiencing chronic heartburn, may be ordered right away to check for the possibility of Barrett's esophagus (see Chapter 6). The acid probe, an ambulatory test (meaning it is conducted on an outpatient basis), is helpful in determining when and how much stomach acid is backwashing your esophagus over a one- to two-day period. Barium x-rays, although used less frequently than in the past because the EGD has become popular, can still be particularly helpful in discovering any narrowing, growths, or the presence of a hiatal hernia.

Is It Hiatal Hernia?

For some patients who are experiencing chronic heartburn and other symptoms of GERD, a hiatal hernia may be the culprit. A hiatal hernia occurs when part of your stomach moves up into the lower chest through a small opening in the diaphragm called the hiatus. If large enough, the hernia can further weaken your LES and worsen any heartburn condition you may already have. Occasionally, surgery is the answer for a large hiatal hernia. If the hernia exerts an exorbitant amount of pressure or is in danger of twisting and cutting off blood supply, it poses an extremely dangerous situation. The most common type of hiatal hernia associated with GERD symptoms is the "sliding" type. In this instance, the sphincter pretty much slips off and abandons its post, leaving the top of the stomach, where acid is produced, with no barrier to acid reflux except for pure gravity.

GI DIDN'T KNOW!

Many people over the age of 50 have a small hiatal hernia simply from the wear and tear of aging, and pregnant women are susceptible to hiatal hernias because of increased abdominal pressure from the growing baby. In most cases, however, surgical treatment is not required because of the increased effectiveness of today's pharmaceuticals.

Allergic Esophagus

Another disorder that can cause symptoms of GERD is a form of eosinophilic gastro-enteritis, an allergic condition that can affect any part of the digestive system. When the esophagus is involved it is called eosinophilic esophagitis or, more familiarly, allergic esophagus. Although still considered rare, allergic esophagus appears to be on the rise, particularly in young adults. Food can become lodged in the esophagus, requiring an endoscopy to remove it or push it through. The patient experiences symptoms of GERD, but the underlying cause is usually difficulty in swallowing.

GI DIDN'T KNOW!

Patients diagnosed with allergic esophagus may have something in common with cats. One specific type of eosinophilic esophagitis, called feline esophagus, is characterized by the appearance of undulating folds or rings in the throat, just like normal kitties have.

An endoscopy with a biopsy is the only way to diagnose allergic esophagus correctly. Your doctor has the biopsied tissue examined for a higher-than-normal presence of allergic-type white blood cells called eosinophils. Once a diagnosis of allergic esophagus is made, you will probably be prescribed allergy medication and be referred to an allergist who conducts skin tests for specific allergens. Once the allergy itself is identified and dealt with through dietary changes and often medication and the difficulty in swallowing has been relieved, your acid reflux symptoms should subside.

Pill Esophagitis

These days Americans are taking more medication than ever. Although most of the time swallowing pills is nothing more than a tedious task, sometimes certain types of drugs actually irritate the esophagus, either on their way down the hatch or by lodging in the lining of the throat, causing symptoms of GERD such as difficulty and pain in swallowing as well as chronic heartburn. When this happens, it is possible to develop a condition called pill esophagitis, also known as drug-induced esophagitis. Your doctor will want to know if you take any potentially esophageal-irritating drugs such as tetracycline, quinidine, or potassium chloride, to name a few, or if you take multiple medications that are in frequent contact with the delicate lining of your esophagus. Often those who don't drink enough fluid when taking pills or who take them right before bedtime are at potential risk for developing pill esophagitis. Drug-induced esophagitis is not an uncommon condition among the elderly and is often seen in nursing homes. Drinking lots of water with medications usually eases the symptoms and allows the esophagus to heal. If GERD symptoms persist, however, your doctor may suggest an alternate drug, or a liquid form of the same drug, in place of the one contributing to your esophagitis. He or she may also recommend short-term use of over-the-counter or prescription medication for relief of your reflux symptoms.

> **TUMMY TIP**
>
> Always take pills with plenty of water—including over-the-counter nonsteroi-dal anti-inflammatory drugs (NSAIDs) such as ibuprofen—to avoid irritation to the esophagus and to prevent the possibility of developing pill esophagitis.

Treating GERD with Medication

Once your doctor has made a diagnosis of acid reflux disease and eliminated any other conditions that might be causing similar symptoms, your treatment begins. Finding the right combination of drug therapy and lifestyle changes that work for you is the goal. However, most lifestyle changes only prove effective in the long term, so a regimen of medication may be necessary to jump-start the program and offer immediate relief of your GERD symptoms. You also don't want to risk any further damage to the esophagus, which could lead to unwanted complications.

Chances are that the usual antacids you've been chomping on when heartburn hits are providing little relief; otherwise, you wouldn't be visiting your doctor in the first place. Long-term use of antacids for short-term relief is not a good idea anyway, as it could result in some unpleasant side effects such as diarrhea or constipation and may even interfere with other medications you take. If you've been diagnosed with GERD, you're probably ready for something more effective.

Antagonizing Acid Reflux

While hunting for antacids at your local drug store, you may have run across acid suppressants known as H-2 blockers in nonprescription form. These are antihistamine-type medications that reduce stomach acid production, providing relief from symptoms of GERD. They specifically block the second of four histamine receptors (thus H-2) in the body known as *parietal cells*. Usually taken before meals and/or at bedtime, H-2 blockers are available in both prescription and nonprescription strengths and are known commercially and generically by names such as Pepcid (famotidine), Tagamet (cimetidine), and Zantac (ranitidine).

> **DEFINITION**
>
> **Parietal cells** are the stomach cells that primarily stimulate gastric acid production.

Unlike antacids that simply neutralize the acid already present, these medications can reduce the amount of acid produced in the first place. Although the effectiveness is not immediate (they take about 30 minutes), it is longer lasting than antacids and may be helpful for mild forms of GERD. Your doctor will want to know if you've tried any nonprescription-strength H-2 blockers, also called antagonists, and received any relief from your symptoms. Because over-the-counter acid reducers are generally half the strength of a prescription H-2 blocker of the same name, a stronger version just might provide the effectiveness you require. In fact, about 60 percent of reflux sufferers receive relief with these types of medications. Normally, a high dose is prescribed at first (for four weeks) and then a lower dose is prescribed afterward for somewhat longer (six to eight weeks). However, if antagonizing your acid reflux disease proves less than successful and you are still experiencing frequent symptoms, it may be time to bring out the big guns and put a halt to acid once and for all.

> **GULP!**
>
> Before embarking on an over-the-counter regimen of H-2 blockers, pregnant women as well as people with symptoms such as weight loss, nausea, vomiting, and bleeding should first consult with their doctors.

Pulling the Plug on Acid

Medications called proton pump inhibitors (PPIs) block the production of acid altogether by shutting down the stomach's natural secretion of acid via the gastric proton pump. This pump is directly responsible for secreting acid into the stomach and is the final stage of the process. Among the most widely sold drugs in the world, PPIs not only relieve GERD symptoms but allow a damaged esophagus to heal. Names of prescribed PPIs you may be familiar with are Prilosec (omeprazole), Prevacid (lanzoprazole), Nexium (esomeprazole), Kapidex (dexlansoprazole), and AcipHex (rabeprazole). Prilosec and Prevacid are also available over the counter for short-term use.

Your doctor may prescribe a PPI for a minimum of three months or for much longer depending on your response. Long-term use (more than six months) is typically safe when required. However, you may have heard about the possibility of your body's levels of vitamin B_{12} being diminished through the use of PPIs, especially in the elderly. This reduction happens because stomach acid is often integral to the absorption of this important vitamin. In reality, however, there are other ways in which B_{12} is absorbed that are not acid dependent, and your body tends to store a good supply of B_{12} anyway (usually several years worth), so B_{12} deficiency is relatively rare.

If blood tests indicate that your B_{12} is in short supply, it may actually be a result of another condition such as pernicious anemia (see Chapter 7). Still, if you are feeling chronically tired, nauseated, tingly in the hands and feet, or even a bit depressed and you are not getting enough B_{12} in your diet (as is often the case with vegetarians who shun animal protein), you may be advised to take a B_{12} supplement. Be sure to mention any B_{12} deficiency symptoms to your doctor whether or not you take a PPI for GERD, particularly if the onset of symptoms coincides with the development of any digestive problems.

Compared to vitamin B_{12}, there is a much greater possibility that calcium absorption may be affected by PPIs. For older adults who have osteoporosis or are at risk for developing it, PPIs could increase the risk of hip fractures, according to a recent study. Calcium supplementation and bone density testing may be recommended for those taking PPIs for an extended period of time in order to combat and avoid this potential risk, and the risk includes any PPIs you may be taking in nonprescription form. Be sure to tell your doctor if this is the case.

GULP!

PPIs may interact with some over-the-counter herbal remedies, as well as medications such as Valium or those taken for epilepsy, blood clot prevention, and nail bed fungus, by either increasing or decreasing their effectiveness. Always let your doctor know about all medications and remedies you are taking.

Another potential, yet relatively infrequent, problem with pulling the plug on acid is that, in the long term, doing so could increase your chances of developing gastrointestinal (GI) infections. Stomach acid normally kills unwanted bacteria, but without it some types of bacteria might flourish. A form of infectious diarrhea, less commonly seen in those taking H-2 blockers, has been associated with PPIs in people over the age of 75, so if you are a senior, your doctor may limit their use. All in all, however, PPIs and their impressive ability to combat and even heal the symptoms of GERD often outweigh their infrequent side effects and risks. Always be sure to consult your doctor, however, if you have any concerns about the long-term use of any medication.

> **GULP!**
>
> For those who cannot tolerate PPIs, surgery for GERD might be recommended, although recently both the long-term effectiveness and danger of such procedures have come into question. Before considering this last resort, be sure you have explored all the pharmaceutical possibilities with your doctor and made a sincere effort to alter your lifestyle.

Treating GERD with Lifestyle Changes

In addition to medication, your doctor will recommend specific changes you can make in your daily life that will reduce and perhaps even eliminate your symptoms of GERD over the long run. The more you are able to make these lifestyle adjustments, the better your chances of reducing acid reflux and preventing future problems.

Take the Pressure Off

We all know that excess weight creates a multitude of health problems, and being overweight or obese has been clearly identified as a major cause of GERD. If you need yet another excuse to shed those pounds, here it is. Extra weight puts pressure on the abdomen and can squish up your internal organs, increasing the likelihood of acid reflux. Whether you're sitting, standing, bending over, or lying down, that excess poundage finds a way to put on the pressure. If you need help jump-starting a diet, ask your doctor for advice. Until the pounds begin to disappear, be cautious about stooping and bending for long periods of time and always loosen your belt (or clothing) if you are feeling particularly constricted, especially after meals.

Make Gravity Work for You

If you experience chronic heartburn or related chest pain when trying to sleep, as most GERD sufferers do, you are probably allowing gravity to work against you. If that esophageal sphincter is weak to begin with, it'll be even more ineffective when you're flat on your back. Elevation is the key, but not with a plumped-up pillow. A scrunched-up neck does nothing for alleviating acid reflux and may actually intensify your symptoms. Instead, raise the head of your bed somewhere between 6 and 9 inches by placing cement or sturdy wooden blocks under the top two legs of the bed frame. Another possibility is to place a wedge between the mattress and box spring at the head of your bed to elevate your body from the waist up. You can purchase these types of wedges at medical supply stores or can rig one up yourself. Performing this small adjustment with gravity will result, for the most part, in keeping acid at bay when you are trying to get some needed sleep and will help to greatly reduce your symptoms of GERD, especially at night.

GI DIDN'T KNOW!

According to the National Sleep Foundation, GERD sufferers are more apt to experience symptoms of sleep disorders such as insomnia, sleep apnea, daytime sleepiness, and restless leg syndrome.

What's That in Your Mouth!

What and how much we consume make a huge difference in combating GERD. Smoking—public enemy number one—plays a notorious role here as everywhere else. In this case, it further weakens that LES, allowing acid to bully its way through. Smoking can also reduce the amount of saliva you produce. Quitting can make a big difference and assists in warding off even more serious conditions such as Barrett's esophagus and cancer. So if you suffer from GERD, saying goodbye to cigarette smoking is a must.

Alcoholic beverages (including wine and beer), in more than moderate amounts and on frequent occasions, can also weaken the esophageal sphincter as well as irritate an inflamed esophagus. Be mindful of your alcohol consumption, particularly at night, and cut back to avoid worsening your GERD. Other beverages that might irritate your esophageal lining and even further weaken the sphincter include fruit juices (especially citrus), coffee and other caffeinated drinks, and carbonated drinks. Be aware that liquid medicines and mouthwash that contain alcohol could irritate the lining, too. Opt for alcohol-free versions whenever possible.

Certain types of foods are known to weaken the esophageal sphincter, so you'll need to cut back or even eliminate these troublemakers. They include chocolate (sorry!), fatty foods, spicy foods, and peppermint. Foods that can cause irritation to a damaged esophagus include onion, garlic, acidic fruits, anything with tomatoes, and peppery spices. Taking vitamin C supplements may also irritate the esophageal lining. Once a good amount of healing has taken place, however, most irritating foods lose their potency, but you should still be cautious when eating them. Keeping a food diary alerts you to specific foods and drinks that seem to affect you personally. Because everyone is a bit different, you may find that something like chocolate might be okay now and again (yay!), particularly once any medication you may be prescribed begins to take effect.

Finally, eating smaller portions of food and avoiding noshing at night can help reduce your GERD woes. It might also help you to shed some weight if that's contributing to your symptoms. The more food there is in your stomach, the more likely the acidic contents will reflux into the esophagus, so try not to overeat. Frequent, smaller meals put less stress on the esophageal sphincter. Ideally, avoid eating between four and six hours before going to bed so that your stomach has a chance to empty partially. By the way, fatty foods and alcohol, in addition to weakening the sphincter, can also delay stomach emptying, as can some medications and conditions such as diabetes.

Don't Stress Me Out

A hectic and stressful lifestyle can definitely contribute to your GERD symptoms. In fact, a recent Gallup poll indicated that 64 percent of GERD sufferers say stress causes their symptoms, particularly heartburn, to worsen. Exactly how this occurs is not entirely known, but it may be connected to a brain-gut mechanism that might increase sensitivity to acid when stress levels rise. Try to manage your stress with leisure activities and relaxation techniques rather than behaviors such as heavy drinking and smoking that only aggravate your symptoms. Learning to relax and chill out are great goals for everyone, but they may be especially important for alleviating immediate GERD symptoms and treating acid reflux for the long term.

Preventing GERD

Now that you know the ins and outs of coping with GERD, including its diagnosis and treatment, you might think that avoiding GERD in the first place may be your best bet. If you experience only occasional heartburn and would like to nip GERD before it creeps up on you, there are important steps you can take right now, especially if you are someone who may be at risk.

More Risky Business

Although you can never be sure whether GERD may be in your future, there are several risk factors—in addition to obesity, poor diet, smoking, and excessive alcohol consumption—that could make it more likely. Eliminating as many of the following factors as you can just might help you stay GERD free.

> **TUMMY TIP**
>
> Don't ignore family history. If someone else in your immediate family, particularly a parent, has been diagnosed with GERD, you may be at a higher risk and should be especially vigilant about other risk factors.

Lack of exercise: Getting up and moving around after a meal is a much better habit to develop than plopping yourself on the sofa. Take a leisurely walk, help with the dishes, or play with the kids. In addition, develop and stick to a regular exercise program doing something you like. It will promote healthier digestion and increase your overall metabolism.

Slow digestion: Some people, particularly diabetics, could be prone to heartburn and other symptoms because of slow digestion, also called delayed gastric emptying. Having a doctor monitor your condition, as well as eating smaller portions, could be important in reducing your risk.

Unmanaged respiratory disease: People with asthma are at very high risk of developing GERD. Those with chronic obstructive pulmonary disease (COPD), which includes chronic bronchitis and emphysema, may also be at risk according to a recent study. The exact connection is not clear, but it could be due to acidic injury to the airways or a nerve reflex that narrows the esophagus to protect the lining when acid begins to rise. Managing your condition with your doctor, taking appropriate medications, and removing triggers that bring on respiratory distress will help to reduce your risk of GERD.

Pregnancy and GERD

One of the greatest risks for developing GERD is being pregnant. This is probably not a risk you are willing to eliminate if you want to start a family. So what can you do to reduce your chances of developing GERD and to help you cope with it if you do?

GERD can occur through several different mechanisms during pregnancy, the most obvious being the additional pressure placed on the stomach area from the growing baby. Hormonal changes, however, can also play a role by slowing the digestive process. Muscles in the esophagus that push food down the pipe also slow down because of hormones, and not only does the LES tend to weaken, it may even open its door when it shouldn't.

Eating a healthy diet in smaller portions and avoiding foods that promote heartburn are some of the dietary precautions you can take. Wearing loose-fitting clothing that doesn't contribute additional pressure to the abdominal area is helpful as well. Antacids are generally safe to use to relieve symptoms when they arise. However, if you are still suffering with severe GERD symptoms, ask your doctor for advice before using any other medications or making any drastic lifestyle changes. The good news is that, most of the time, once the baby is born, symptoms of GERD greatly diminish or disappear entirely.

The Least You Need to Know

- Acid reflux disease, also called GERD, is a disorder in which stomach acid backs up into the esophagus, causing irritation and chronic heartburn.
- Far more serious than occasional heartburn, GERD may result in dangerous complications, including esophageal cancer, if left untreated.
- A diagnosis of GERD is usually made by reporting symptoms to your doctor and, more definitively, through an upper endoscopy.
- Reflux disease is easily treatable with both a variety of medications and long-term lifestyle changes.
- You can reduce your chances of developing acid reflux disease by lowering or eliminating your risk factors.

Barrett's Esophagus and Esophageal Cancer

In This Chapter

- The risks of disregarding GERD
- Barrett's esophagus and changes in cell tissue
- The aggressive nature of esophageal cancer

The last chapter looked at acid reflux disease and its probable causes, as well as the types of lifestyle changes and medications normally recommended to keep it under control. With good medical attention and strict follow-through, acid reflux disease, or gastrointestinal reflux disease (GERD), can be addressed without a great amount of concern. In fact, if you are diligent about making improvements to your life, such as weight loss, stress reduction, and more exercise, you'll probably start feeling better than you've felt in quite some time. Eating healthier, smaller meals at proper times of the day also has a dramatic effect on your condition and contributes to better health overall.

However, be aware that GERD, when ignored and untreated, can only get worse. In this chapter, we'll look at the potentially serious results that might occur if GERD is left unchecked. Unfortunately, it is also true that, in some cases, despite treatment or even a history of acid reflux, some people may be predisposed to the possibility of more serious esophageal diseases such as Barrett's esophagus or cancer. We'll look at who is at highest risk and what can be done to prevent further damage to the esophagus.

Although esophageal cancer and Barrett's esophagus are usually discussed together, it is not a foregone conclusion that all people who suffer from Barrett's will eventually be stricken with cancer. In reality, at present only between 5 and 10 percent of

Barrett's sufferers go on to develop esophageal cancer. In addition, there are other risk factors besides Barrett's that may cause cancer of the esophagus. We'll look at those factors as we examine the diagnostic procedures, treatments, and therapies that are available once suspicion of either of these conditions arises.

> **GI DIDN'T KNOW!**
>
> Barrett's esophagus is named for the Australian surgeon Norman Barrett, who first described this condition in 1957.

When GERD Gets Serious

GERD is characterized by inflammation of the esophagus and is accompanied by symptoms such as excessive belching, persistent heartburn, and chest pain, among other probable symptoms (see Chapter 5). Between 5 and 15 percent of people who seek help for their symptoms of GERD are actually diagnosed with Barrett's esophagus. Barrett's esophagus is a condition in which cells of the esophagus change in response to their exposure to acid. Many patients whose tests reveal that Barrett's is present, however, do not experience symptoms at all. It is believed that the majority of people who are insensitive to typical GERD manifestations of heartburn, soreness, and chest pain are ultimately more likely to develop Barrett's esophagus because GERD goes unchecked. Ironically, GERD symptoms often subside once Barrett's is present because the change in cells makes the esophagus more able to handle the acid.

An Identity Crisis

The cells that line the esophagus are delicate in nature, which is why stomach acid so easily irritates the lining when reflux occurs. After chronic exposure to acid, the esophageal lining may actually begin to change in order to adapt. Through a process called *metaplasia*, a change takes place in the lower part of the esophagus near the stomach. To protect the esophagus, cells transform into stomach lining cells, which are better equipped to cope with acid. This change may explain, in part, why Barrett's sufferers often lack typical symptoms of GERD. Eventually, the stomach cells lining the esophagus change yet again into cells similar to those in the small intestine lining, a trademark of Barrett's. These changes are the reason why physicians refer to Barrett's esophagus by the more technical term "intestinal metaplasia of the esophagus." Once cell changes begin, by the way, they continue on a path of change. Intestinal cells can become precancerous, and these cells, in turn, can develop into cancer.

DEFINITION

Metaplasia is the changing of one specialized cell into another specialized cell, usually because of an abnormal stimulus.

State of Change

With the change in cells, a color change also takes place. Light pink esophageal cells turn salmon in color, a change usually visible by your doctor with an upper endoscope. Other symptoms that may or may not be present with Barrett's include the following:

- Persistent acid reflux disease symptoms
- Vomiting of blood
- Black or bloody stool
- Unexplained weight loss

Who's at Risk?

Barrett's esophagus affects about 1 percent of the population, and those who have had reflux disease for 5 to 10 years are definitely at greater risk. In addition, there are other factors that can contribute to a higher risk of developing Barrett's. Men are twice as likely as women to be diagnosed, and Caucasian people appear to be more susceptible than other races. Individuals who have had some type of ulceration in the esophagus, a stricture, or narrowing of the esophagus due to other conditions besides GERD, may be predisposed to Barrett's. Those who suffer from bile reflux or hiatal hernia may also be at a higher risk.

Age is also a factor. People over 45 are at a higher risk than those who are younger. However, Barrett's can often go undetected for many years, so it is possible that a percentage of people in a lower age bracket are also at risk. Still, the average age of diagnosis is 50, so it is safe to assume that this disease is not a common one among younger people. Indeed, it is an extremely rare condition in children.

GULP!

As with GERD, heavy alcohol intake and smoking can be contributing factors to Barrett's. In fact, people who both smoke and drink to excess are at an even greater risk for developing esophageal diseases because one appears to increase the adverse effects of the other.

Getting a Diagnosis

Because of the potential lack of symptoms, many doctors recommend that patients between the ages of 40 and 50 with a history of chronic acid reflux disease be examined for Barrett's. The only way to obtain a diagnosis is through an upper gastrointestinal (GI) endoscopy (see Chapter 5) and biopsy. If the esophageal tissue looks suspect, the doctor removes several small pieces during the endoscopic procedure. Tissue from this biopsy is processed and examined by a pathologist. Using the results of the biopsy and the general results of your endoscopy, your gastroenterologist can make a diagnosis.

> **GI DIDN'T KNOW!**
>
> In rare instances, an area of stomach tissue called an inlet patch can grow in the upper part of the esophagus. This condition also warrants watching, although it rarely becomes cancerous.

Initial Treatment

Recent studies have shown that treating Barrett's esophagus with proton pump inhibitors (PPIs; see Chapter 5), like those prescribed for acid reflux disease, can diminish the risk of progression to esophageal cancer. If you are not already taking a form of this medication, your doctor will almost surely prescribe one. Lifestyle changes must definitely be made. Once Barrett's esophagus has been diagnosed, it is doubly imperative that these changes, similar to many of the recommendations for treating GERD, be made. These lifestyle changes include the following:

- Quitting smoking
- Substituting for nitrates, calcium channel blockers, and certain asthma medications that can weaken the lower esophageal sphincter (LES)
- Avoiding foods and beverages that weaken the LES such as chocolate, peppermint, fatty foods, coffee, and alcohol
- Avoiding foods and beverages that irritate the esophagus such as citrus fruits and juices, tomato products, and pepper
- Reducing portion sizes of meals
- Not eating late at night

- Getting up and moving around after eating

- Elevating the head of the bed (see Chapter 5)

- Avoiding unnecessary pressure on the abdomen caused by bending, lifting, or the wearing of tight clothing

TUMMY TIP

There is new evidence that drugs called COX II inhibitors, such as Celebrex, may play a role in preventing progression to esophageal cancer. Many concerns surrounding this medication exist, however, so it should be taken only under the supervision of your doctor.

Under Surveillance

One of the most important aspects of your treatment is continued surveillance of the esophagus. You must undergo an upper GI endoscopy and biopsy every year or two to check for signs of *dysplasia*. This condition would indicate the development of precancerous cells, which are evaluated to determine whether they are low- or high-grade changes. Low-grade dysplasia will be monitored with endoscopies and biopsies for any progression. High-grade dysplasia, however, may be treated with surgery and/or other therapies. Before a definitive diagnosis of high-grade or severe dysplasia is made, two pathologists must confirm the findings because of the high stakes involved.

DEFINITION

Dysplasia is the earliest form of a precancerous condition and indicates an abnormal development or growth in an organ, tissue, or cell.

Treating Severe Changes

When there is evidence that high-grade dysplasia has occurred, on rare occasions your doctor may recommend a type of endoscopic treatment or actual surgery in order to ward off the progression to cancer. Be sure you understand all the available options and the potential risks and benefits of each. Remember that not all patients diagnosed with Barrett's at the high-grade level will develop cancer and can continue to be monitored for years. If you are having difficulty in making an educated decision, do not hesitate to seek another opinion or inquire further with any medical professionals who may have extensive experience in this area.

Endoscopic Therapies

Several different endoscopic therapies are available to treat Barrett's esophagus. During these therapies, the Barrett's lining is destroyed and the dysplasia removed. The ultimate goal is to encourage the growth of normal esophageal tissue where the Barrett's tissue once was. Most therapies are used on their own but on occasion may be used together.

During photodynamic therapy (PDT), the patient receives an injection of a light-sensitive drug that makes all the cells in the body hypersensitive to light exposure. This sensitivity requires a bit of time to take effect. After about 48 hours, the patient returns for the actual endoscopic procedure. A laser light is passed through the endoscope and is used to destroy the Barrett's cells. Complications may include chest pain, nausea, and sun sensitivity for several weeks.

Another therapy, called an endoscopic mucosal resection (EMR), mostly used in treating cancer, is occasionally employed for Barrett's. It involves lifting the offending lining through an endoscope and, by applying suction on a saline injected area, cutting it off and removing it back out through the endoscope. Complications can include esophageal bleeding or tears to the lining.

Finally, thermal *ablation* may be used to destroy Barrett's cells by burning them off with an electrical probe, laser, or gas. Halo ablation has recently become a popular therapy as well, which, in a strange way, during the procedure, resembles the marks you get on raw chicken when placed on a hot grill. Later the esophagus looks normal. Other therapies that involve freezing or radio frequency ablation are presently being explored for effectiveness. The danger with most of these techniques is that they may create "buried Barrett's" as new tissue covers up the old, making it impossible to see and ultimately biopsy.

DEFINITION

Ablation refers to the surgical removal of body tissue or a part of the body and comes from the Latin word meaning "to carry off."

Surgery as a Solution

One type of surgery sometimes recommended for Barrett's sufferers is called Nissen fundoplication, often referred to as antireflux surgery. Occasionally performed on patients with acid reflux disease who cannot tolerate medication, this surgery can be performed by a skilled surgeon in a *laparoscopic* procedure that is minimally invasive. During the surgery, a portion of the upper stomach is wrapped around the esophagus and stitched in place, strengthening a weakened LES and keeping stomach acid from rising. Although the procedure doesn't actually treat Barrett's esophagus in a true sense, it prevents further acid exposure that could result in precancerous cell changes. Rare complications include esophageal motility problems (due to tightening of the sphincter) such as difficulty swallowing or an inability to belch or vomit.

DEFINITION

Laparoscopic surgery is a technique in which small incisions are made in the abdominal area, where a camera and instruments are inserted to perform operations. Laparoscopic surgery is most commonly used in gallbladder removal.

When Barrett's esophagus has reached high-grade dysplasia, on occasion an esophagectomy, removal of all or part of the esophagus, is recommended to avoid cancer. Normally more often seen for cancer sufferers, this treatment, although somewhat controversial in today's age of technology, is still the norm for Barrett's with high-grade dysplasia.

Finding Benign Tumors

Although rare, it is possible to have tumor growth in the esophagus that is not cancerous. These benign (noncancerous) growths do not often produce symptoms, but on occasion their presence may cause symptoms such as difficulty or pain in swallowing or regurgitation of stomach contents. They are more common in men than in women and do not usually appear until a person is beyond the age of 40.

Leiomyoma and Polyps

Smooth, projecting growths on the lining of the esophagus are called leiomyomas and are the most common of the benign tumors. More than half the people who have them experience no symptoms at all, and unless they interfere with swallowing, they are not usually removed. Often detected during a barium x-ray or endoscopy, most leiomyomas are located in the lower third of the esophagus. About 80 percent of esophageal polyps, however, are found in the upper area of the esophagus near the pharynx. These are the second-most-common benign tumors of the esophagus and, like leiomyomas, do not often create symptoms. In some instances, a patient may feel as if there is a lump in the throat or may experience a bit of regurgitation. However, in rare and extreme cases, some polyps could be regurgitated and cut off air supply, causing choking or even death. In cases with this risk, surgical removal would be necessary.

Papillomas and Granular Cell Tumors

Lesions known as squamous cell papillomas are sometimes found in the esophagus at the back, lower area. They are usually quite small and may be discovered during an upper endoscopy. Often caused by the HPV virus associated with genital warts (one direct cause of cervical cancer), these lesions can be a risk factor for cancer of the esophagus.

Granular cell tumors, more often seen on the tongue, can sometimes appear in the esophagus. Rarely do they grow very large, and unless they present any symptoms, they are not surgically removed. Very rarely, granular cell tumors may actually be malignant (cancerous) and not benign.

Esophageal Cancer—Who's at Risk?

There are two common types of esophageal cancer, each carrying its own risk factors. Acid reflux disease and Barrett's esophagus are generally the precursors to adenocarcinoma, a cancer that originates in glandular tissue. Squamous cell *carcinoma* arises from the cells lining the upper esophagus and has a number of risk factors connected with it. *Squamous cell cancer* is also the more common of the two worldwide, mainly occurring in Asian males.

DEFINITION

Carcinoma is any malignant cancer of tissue cells. **Squamous cell cancer** is a form of carcinoma that can occur at the beginning of the esophagus and the end of the colon but which is most commonly seen on the skin.

Common Factors

In general, both carcinomas are usually seen in adults over the age of 60 and are more likely in men than women. However, specific factors increase the risk of esophageal cancer for anyone:

- Heredity
- Tobacco smoking
- Heavy alcohol consumption
- Obesity
- Celiac disease
- Swallowing disorders
- Swallowing lye or other caustic substances

Limited research has shown that esophageal cancer has possible connections to human papillomavirus (HPV), chemical compounds called nitrosamines (similar to nitrates), radiation therapy to the upper chest area, and even a high consumption of extremely hot beverages. Individuals with a history of cancers to the neck or head area are at a clear risk for developing esophageal cancer.

Decreased Risk?

There is some evidence that certain things we consume may actually decrease our chances of developing esophageal cancer. Moderate coffee drinking has been associated with a lower risk, as has a diet high in cruciferous vegetables such as cabbage, broccoli, and cauliflower. Eating plenty of green- and yellow-colored vegetables and fruits may also be protective.

GI DIDN'T KNOW!

A debatable but delicious Italian study showed that eating pizza more than twice a week decreased the chances of all digestive-related cancers, including esophageal, among the Italian population.

Similarly, regular use of aspirin or nonsteroidal anti-inflammatory drugs (NSAIDs) such as ibuprofen may decrease the risk of cancer of the esophagus, but because of their many risks, they should not be taken as a preventive measure.

Diagnosis and Staging

Early detection of esophageal cancer can be difficult because often there are no significant symptoms to investigate. Unless you are under surveillance for Barrett's esophagus, you may not undergo any testing that could reveal the cancer's presence. When symptoms finally appear, they are often similar to acid reflux disease and may simply be treated with medication without an upper GI endoscopy. It is only through an upper GI endoscopy and biopsy, however, that esophageal cancer can be diagnosed.

If you experience the typical symptoms of acid reflux disease (see Chapter 5) and also note any of the following, you should consult your doctor immediately:

- Severe weight loss

- Pain in the throat or back

- Pain between the shoulder blades

- Chronic coughing or hoarseness

- Vomiting

- Coughing up blood

- Lodging of food in the throat

Location and Spread

Once the proper preliminary testing is conducted and a diagnosis of esophageal cancer is made, your doctor zeroes in on the location and determines whether the cancer has spread to any other parts of your body. Location and biopsy results indicate the type of esophageal cancer that is present—adenocarcinoma or squamous cell carcinoma. The esophagus is commonly divided into three sections in order to make it easier to discuss location, and the tumor location is measured by its distance from the teeth to one of these three sections.

Esophageal cancer tends to be more aggressive than some other digestive system cancers because there is one less layer in the esophagus than in the stomach for the cancer to penetrate to spread outside the organ. The first place to which esophageal cancer normally spreads is the lymph nodes, little bean-shaped parts of the immune system. However, cancer can *metastasize* to almost any other part of the body as well, so further testing is required. Your doctor may perform any of the following to investigate other areas that may be affected:

- Computed tomography (CT) scans provide detailed pictures of the chest, abdomen, and pelvis to check for any spread to vital organs, particularly to the liver. Its sensitivity is limited to the detection of masses, however.

- Endoscopic ultrasounds (EUS) of the esophagus reveal any spread to nearby lymph nodes and have become commonplace in staging the cancer.

- Positron emission tomography (PET) scans give a better view of lymph nodes and help determine the cause of any abnormal size.

- Bone scans using radioactive substances injected into the veins can show abnormal bone growth.

DEFINITION

A cancer is said to **metastasize** when it has spread from one organ to another nonadjacent organ or part of the body, usually through the lymphatic system or bloodstream.

Classification by Stages

It is vitally important to know the degree to which cancer has progressed, as well as its level of aggressiveness, in order to determine an appropriate treatment plan. Identifying the situation is called staging and is generally categorized with four levels. Sometimes a "Stage 0" is used to indicate the presence of abnormal cells in the innermost lining of the esophagus, also referred to as carcinoma in situ. However, the following stages (including some substages) are the classifications most commonly used:

> **Stage I:** Cancer cells have spread from the innermost lining to the next layer of tissue in the wall of the esophagus.

> **Stage II:** This stage is divided into two levels, depending on where the cancer has spread.

>> **Stage IIA:** Cancer has spread to the esophageal muscle or outer wall.

>> **Stage IIB:** Cancer may have spread to any of the three layers and also to nearby lymph nodes.

> **Stage III:** Cancer has spread to the outer wall and possibly nearby tissue or lymph nodes.

Stage IV: This stage is divided into two levels, like Stage II.

Stage IVA: Cancer has spread to nearby or distant lymph nodes.

Stage IVB: Cancer has spread to distant lymph nodes and/or other organs.

Treating Esophageal Cancer

By far the most common form of treatment is to surgically remove the tumor or part of the esophagus. In a partial esophagectomy, a portion of the stomach is pulled up and joined to the healthy remaining esophagus. Occasionally a plastic tube or part of the intestine is used to form the connection. In some cases a total esophagectomy may be necessary, in which case the stomach takes the place of the esophagus or another hollow structure is used such as part of the colon.

> **GULP!**
>
> Many patients, either from the cancer itself or as a result of treatment, find it difficult to eat and obtain nourishment. Intravenous feeding or the placement of a feeding tube into the stomach may be necessary until patients can comfortably eat on their own.

Surgery of this magnitude on the esophagus is very likely to cause short-term pain and discomfort in the chest area. Medication helps to control pain, while special breathing and coughing techniques taught by a physical therapist make recovery a bit easier. Both major and minor complications from an esophagectomy are possible and can occur in nearly 40 percent of cases. Recovery time in the hospital is normally one to two weeks, with a total recovery time from a few months to up to a year in some instances. In general, however, lifelong recovery is the norm, as this type of surgery changes one's way of life in very noticeable ways.

Combination Therapies

A team of specialists joins the gastroenterologist in treating a patient's esophageal cancer. The team includes medical and radiation oncologists, a surgeon, therapists, and possibly a nutritionist or other type of specialist. Together with a specific treatment plan designed for every individual, different therapy treatments are conducted in combination or one after another. Studies show that administering multiple therapies increases the survival rate for esophageal cancer. These therapies include the following:

- Chemotherapy before and/or after surgery

- Radiation before or in place of surgery

- Laser therapy to relieve blockages

- Electrocoagulation to destroy cancer cells

New treatments undergo clinical testing, and it is worth finding out if there are any clinical trials in which you may be qualified to participate. Ask your doctor and check with the National Institutes of Health as well as hospitals specializing in cancer treatment (see Appendix B).

Follow-Up Care

Survival rates for esophageal cancer are generally not promising, mainly because of the advanced stage at which most cancers are discovered. Indeed, esophageal cancer has one of the lowest survival rates of all cancers. If discovered at Stage I or II, however, the three-year survival rate has recently been put at 40 percent when combination therapies are used.

Once a diagnosis of any cancer is made, careful follow-up is of extreme importance. Many of the tests done before surgery may continue to be done after surgery at strategic intervals to check for a recurrence or the effect of treatment. This type of follow-up should continue for the rest of your life so that any changes can be investigated immediately and treated promptly if necessary.

The Least You Need to Know

- Ten percent of GERD patients develop Barrett's esophagus.
- In some patients, Barrett's can be a precursor of esophageal cancer and should be closely monitored.
- Treatment therapies are recommended when high-grade dysplasia is present in Barrett's esophagus.
- Esophageal cancer has of two main types, and some people may be at greater risk for one or the other.
- Surgery, together with radiation therapy, is the most common treatment for esophageal cancer.
- Combination therapies for esophageal cancer can increase survival rates.

Gastritis and Ulcer Disease

In This Chapter

- The inflammation connection to gastric disorders
- *H. pylori* and ulcers
- Serious diseases of the stomach

In exploring the causes, diagnosis, and treatment of gastritis and ulcer disease, it's time to move on from the esophagus and take a closer look at another digestive team player—the stomach. As we learned in Chapter 2, this digestive organ can be pretty tough and hard working as well. Shaped a bit like the letter "J" and situated in your upper-left abdominal cavity, the stomach is responsible for processing the food you eat by breaking it down through churning, grinding, and liquefying.

Although the stomach lining itself is pretty robust, it can still become damaged. Your stomach also produces a type of mucous barrier during digestion in order to protect the stomach wall from harsh exposure to acid. In addition, special blood flow to the stomach lining keeps it happy, a process that can go wrong with severe stress such as from a car accident, job, or relationship problem. When the balance of these mechanisms is off kilter, irritation in the stomach occurs, and eventually gastritis or ulcer disease can result. We now know that these disorders, once believed to be caused strictly from food or stress, have different and far more specific roots. We'll be looking at those causes in detail during our discussion.

Because the stomach is such a remarkably staunch organ, we are often not aware of any irritation or inflammation until symptoms become serious. For this reason, gastritis and ulcer disease can be tricky to diagnose in their early stages. In this chapter, we'll take a look at potential symptoms, ways in which diagnoses may be obtained, and what kinds of treatment are available for those with these tummy-related disorders. We'll also look briefly at some serious stomach occurrences, including pernicious anemia and gastric cancer.

I Can't Stomach This

Mistakenly, many people think that gastritis means excess gas. Although bloating and belching may be experienced by some, gastritis is actually defined as an inflammation of the stomach lining. This inflammation can be attributed to a number of factors, but more often than not, it is caused by either long-term (and sometimes short-term) use of nonsteroidal anti-inflammatory drugs (NSAIDs) such as aspirin and ibuprofen, or infection from bacteria known as *Helicobacter pylori* or *H. pylori*. In both instances, the protective mucous barrier of the stomach is damaged, making the stomach lining more vulnerable to acid and inflammation.

A Colony of Bacteria

The discovery and acknowledgement of *H. pylori* has had a significant effect on the way the medical community now views, diagnoses, and treats most gastric and duodenum (upper small bowel) disorders. It is believed that up to half of the world's population carries these bacteria in their upper GI tracts, where they colonize in the deeper layers of the stomach's lining. Once there, they pretty much set up shop and stay for the remainder of your life. Although stomach acid can kill many types of bacteria, *H. pylori* produces an acid-neutralizing enzyme that allows it to live in an acidic environment where it continues to thrive and sets up a chronic inflammatory response from the immune system. The body still recognizes these bacteria as foreign, so it reacts with an immune system inflammatory response. Interestingly, the nature of this reaction varies from person to person.

GI DIDN'T KNOW!

In 1994, the World Health Organization classified *H. pylori* as a group 1 carcinogen. Group 1 carcinogens cause cancer in humans.

Surprisingly, and for reasons that are still unclear, many people infected with *H. pylori* who develop gastritis manage to live in reasonable harmony with it, absent any symptoms. This situation doesn't mean that there is no damage done, however. Chronic infection can still lead to disorders and even stomach cancer. Still, only a minority of people have symptoms from their gastritis or end up with ulcer disease or cancer. There may be a genetic role at play as well as a factor of contagion. Exposure plays a role, too, as sewage workers, followed by gastroenterologists and GI nurses, appear to be at the top of the list for susceptibility in the workplace. Infection often takes place in childhood, but adults can become infected as well. Until recently, *H. pylori* was relatively rare in the United States, but with increasing globalization, the bacteria have most definitely increased by leaps and bounds.

I Can't Stomach That Either

In addition to prolonged use of NSAIDs and the presence of *H. pylori*, other factors can contribute to the development of gastritis and ulcer disease. These factors include the following:

- **Substance abuse or dependence:** Nicotine, alcohol, and illicit drugs such as cocaine can decrease the protective effect of the mucous barrier.

- **Illness, injuries, and stress:** These can increase acid production, slow digestion, and change the protective blood flow.

- **Heredity and age:** Family history as well as ethnicity (Hispanic, Native American, African American, Asian) and natural aging can have an effect.

- **Bile reflux:** Bile moving from the small intestine back into the stomach may be a factor.

- **Immune system disorders:** Antibodies attacking the stomach lining can cause inflammation.

- **Inflammatory bowel disease (IBD):** Although normally affecting the intestines, IBD in the form of Crohn's disease (CD) can also on occasion affect the stomach.

- **Steroid use:** These drugs, when used in combination with NSAIDs, can actually increase the risk of ulcer disease tenfold.

Symptoms and Diagnosis of Gastritis

Gastritis is usually classified as acute or chronic. Acute gastritis, the more serious, tends to come on suddenly, whereas chronic gastritis may not be felt at all. Although symptoms can often be absent in both cases, when they do appear they are usually experienced as abdominal pain and upset. Sometimes there is bloating or a feeling of fullness as well as belching, nausea, and perhaps vomiting. There may also be a burning sensation or gnawing pain in the upper abdomen. The intestines may be affected, especially if the immune system is weak, and it is also possible to get some degree of viral infection.

GULP!

Gastritis can result in bleeding of the stomach. Signs of blood in the stool or the vomiting of blood require immediate medical attention.

Simple Solutions

Gastritis is extremely common, and in most cases people recover without much more than a few simple alterations in diet and lifestyle. Relating your symptoms and evaluating your medical history may be enough for your gastroenterologist to make a diagnosis of gastritis and prescribe treatment. In general, mild cases of gastritis that flare up from time to time can easily be kept at bay by eliminating triggers that appear to cause symptoms. These triggers might be things such as alcohol, aspirin or other medications, cigarette smoking, or caffeinated beverages. With these triggers gone, the stomach lining often heals on its own within a brief period.

Switching from regular aspirin to an enteric-coated one that does not dissolve in the stomach is a possible solution for some, although this approach is subject to some debate. If NSAIDs are the cause, substituting an acetaminophen such as Tylenol could provide relief. Taking medication on a full stomach or with an antacid may help as well. Your doctor may even go ahead and prescribe a histamine (H-2) blocker or a proton pump inhibitor (PPI; see Chapter 5), medications used to treat acid reflux disease, to reduce acid production in the stomach. A PPI may actually be helpful in negating the effects of NSAIDs, although this should be done under a doctor's supervision.

GULP!

Always consult your doctor before treating any condition with acetaminophen-type drugs such as Tylenol because severe liver damage and even fatal over-dosing has been known to occur, especially in people who drink alcohol on a regular basis.

Tummy Tests

Often, after hearing your symptoms, your gastroenterologist may wish to perform an upper GI endoscopy and take a tissue sample that ultimately reveals the facts, often by eliminating the presence of other disorders or conditions. By looking closely at the lining of your stomach, your doctor can note clear signs of inflammation including redness and swelling, as well as any possible progression toward ulcer disease. Blood and stool tests may also be conducted. A urea breath test (see Chapter 4), which will be instrumental once treatment for *H. pylori* has begun—if that is the cause of your gastritis—may also be done at this time.

GI DIDN'T KNOW!

For reasons yet unknown, redness of the stomach lining can sometimes be caused by depression.

Treating *H. pylori* Infection

If your doctor diagnoses *H. pylori* infection as the cause of your gastritis, treatment involves a number of approaches. Because *H. pylori* is a bacterial infection, it will need to be eradicated through the administration of antibiotics. A combination drug therapy is most likely in order to cope with your gastritis symptoms and to assist the healing process while the antibiotics work.

TUMMY TIP

During your treatment for gastritis, the doctor may suggest a bland diet. Eliminating things that could cause stomach upset, such as spicy dishes, acidic beverages, and fried or fatty foods, may help reduce pain and promote healing.

An Antibiotic Regimen

Two types of antibiotics, taken together, make up the regimen you are likely to receive. For those who are not allergic to penicillin, the combination may include amoxicillin and clarithromycin. Metronidazole might replace the amoxicillin if penicillin is not used. In addition, your doctor may prescribe a PPI such as Prilosec as well in order to control acid production. PPIs also seem to have the added benefit of inhibiting *H. pylori* activity. Bismuth, the active ingredient in medications such as Pepto-Bismol, seems to be able to thwart *H. pylori* activity, too, so bismuth may also be included in your treatment plan. The regimen is usually taken for one to two weeks, with a follow-up urea breath test about eight weeks afterward to check for any lingering *H. pylori* bacteria.

Antibiotic Resistance

Unfortunately, there is a growing occurrence of antibiotic-resistant bacteria, and *H. pylori* are no exception. In fact, it appears that an increased number of people infected with *H. pylori* are harboring a resistant form that may cause initial treatment to fail. In these cases, additional rounds of antibiotics or switching to different ones may be necessary. In the future, a vaccine may be an option as well.

It has been suggested that *H. pylori* bacteria may actually be normal flora, or micro-organisms, of the stomach with potential benefits. A primitive type of bacteria, *H. pylori* may have once assisted in reducing the occurrence of acid reflux and even diseases such as type 2 diabetes and asthma, conditions that have become more prevalent since modern medicine has targeted and successfully eradicated *H. pylori* in many individuals. Further study may ultimately prove that this is the case.

Atrophic Gastritis

Chronic inflammation of the stomach can sometimes result in tissue destruction of the protective mucosal lining—a form of *atrophy*. Atrophic gastritis can lead to the loss of certain important gastric cells and the replacement of them with intestinal-type tissue, a direct precursor to gastric cancer. The stomach's secretion of digestive juices is greatly impaired, contributing to other serious digestive problems and even anemia.

> **DEFINITION**
>
> **Atrophy** is the wasting away of tissue or body parts caused by a number of factors including disease and disuse.

Automatic Response?

Atrophic gastritis is usually caused either by persistent infection from *H. pylori* bacteria (type B gastritis) or an autoimmune response of the body (type A gastritis). When *H. pylori* or dietary factors are the cause, this form of gastritis is said to be environmental in nature, although it is believed that *H. pylori* may trigger an auto-immune response as well. Each type results in its own distinct tissue changes, so a biopsy can determine which of the two you may have, along with other tests for *H. pylori.*

> **GI DIDN'T KNOW!**
>
> Atrophic gastritis/pernicious anemia is the most common autoimmune dis-order that can develop in patients with Graves' disease, another autoimmune disorder involving the thyroid.

Pernicious Anemia

Type A gastritis (autoimmune) can result in a condition known as pernicious anemia. An essential substance called intrinsic factor, which is necessary for the absorption of vitamin B_{12}, is greatly reduced along with stomach acid and enzymes. A deficiency of this essential vitamin, which can only be obtained through diet, results in subsequent anemia. Determining whether pernicious anemia is present can be tricky, although extensive blood tests, including a check for antibodies, usually result in a diagnosis. Supplements that require digestion are no help because the digestive process is disrupted. However, injections of B_{12} as well as nasal supplements help to replenish the supply.

Peptic Ulcer Disease

Ulcer disease, also known as peptic ulcer disease (PUD), is the condition of having an ulcer in the stomach or duodenum (upper small bowel). The word "peptic" refers to the digestive enzyme pepsin, which along with acid secretion aids in digestion. We've all heard people remark "I must have an ulcer," when they experience burning in the abdomen after eating, but unless diagnosed, they may be mistaken. Severe heartburn or gastritis could be the culprit. Often, people who actually have ulcers don't even know it because there may be no symptoms present or only a vague sense of pain.

> **DEFINITION**
>
> An **ulcer** is a break or chronic sore in the lining of the stomach or duodenum. Ulcers can form in areas exposed to gastric acid and pepsin.

Erosion at Work

Problems arise when the stomach lining begins to break down as a result of disruption of the delicate balance of acid and protective mucous. Unlike the mere inflammation of gastritis, erosion of the lining begins to take place, and this erosion is the first step toward the formation of ulcers. As with gastritis, however, the main causes of erosion are prolonged use of NSAIDs or the presence of *H. pylori* bacteria. In fact, it is believed that NSAIDs account for about 25 percent of eventual gastric ulcers, while the remaining 75 percent are usually caused by *H. pylori*. In some instances, people may secrete an excess of gastric acid that can also result in ulcers.

GI DIDN'T KNOW!

Men and women are about equally vulnerable to gastritis, but men appear to be twice as likely to develop ulcers.

Types of Ulcers

The majority of ulcers occur in the stomach or duodenum, in which case they are referred to as a gastric ulcer or a duodenal ulcer. On occasion, ulcers also occur in the esophagus. Contrary to popular belief, most peptic ulcers are of the duodenal type and are almost always benign. Gastric ulcers are less common and may, in some cases, need to be checked for malignancy.

Ulcers appear as craterlike sores and are usually about ¼ to ¾ inch in diameter, although they can also be up to 1 or 2 inches wide. Once erosion has begun, stomach juices—acid and pepsin—go to work on the damaged lining as if to "digest" it, resulting in the typical sore or ulcer with which we are familiar. Whether gastric or duodenal, bleeding or perforation of the lining can take place.

In general, although not always, gastric ulcers cause abdominal pain after eating, while pain from duodenal ulcers is often relieved by eating. These symptoms are among the important facts you need to communicate to your doctor. Ulcers in the stomach usually hit people over the age of 40 who have a history of aspirin or NSAID use for arthritis. Duodenal ulcers appear to affect a younger group between 20 and 40 years of age and are almost always due to *H. pylori*.

GULP!

Excess alcohol consumption and smoking do not directly cause ulcers, although these habits may contribute to their formation and will no doubt affect the success of any treatment a patient receives.

Symptoms and Complications of Ulcer Disease

Although signs of peptic ulcer disease may not initially appear, certain symptoms are associated with their presence and should be noted when speaking with your doctor. They include the following:

- Pain below the rib cage on the left or right

- Abdominal bloating

- *Waterbrash*

- Nausea, vomiting, or vomiting of blood

- Loss of appetite and weight loss

- Dark, foul-smelling stool

DEFINITION

Waterbrash is the flooding of the mouth with saliva, usually after a severe heartburn episode or acidic regurgitation. It is a symptom of peptic ulcer disease as well as GERD.

Ulcers that do not present symptoms are sometimes called silent ulcers. They are most common in older adults, people with diabetes, and those who use NSAIDs.

Bleeding Ulcers

Untreated ulcers can result in bleeding. If an ulcer happens to erode into a blood vessel, major arterial bleeding can occur, requiring immediate attention and even surgery. But slow-bleeding ulcers can be just as troublesome, as they often continue because of the lack of apparent symptoms. Eventually, fatigue, lightheadedness, and shortness of breath can develop from resulting anemia, and vomiting of blood or the passing of dark stool may arise.

Although an upper GI endoscopy often provides a definitive diagnosis, your doctor, upon hearing your symptoms, may use other tests if he or she suspects bleeding. A fecal occult blood test (FOBT) as well as a complete blood count (CBC; see Chapter 4) can also shed light and help your physician put the pieces together for a proper diagnosis. An endoscopy, however, can often be the ideal tool because it not only diagnoses and locates the ulcer, it may also allow your doctor to treat the ulcer at the same time. Treatment is performed by cauterizing or burning a leaking blood vessel at the exact location. Further treatment includes a PPI prescription, dietary changes such as those for gastritis, and follow-up exams.

Emergency Perforations

Occasionally an ulcer can eat right through the stomach or duodenal wall, causing what is known as a perforation or perforated ulcer. Digestive juices and food leach into the abdominal cavity and create a surgical emergency. If untreated, peritonitis—an inflammation of the abdominal cavity wall—can occur, leading to a dangerous infection. X-rays can check for the presence of air in the abdominal cavity, and a computed tomography (CT) scan provides further information. Usually, however, when all symptoms point to severe perforation, surgery takes place immediately because the condition is often life threatening.

Gastric Tumors and Cancer

Various types of growths, including tumors, can develop from the layers of the stomach lining, and most of the time these tumors are benign. Small tumors rarely cause any symptoms at all and are usually found accidentally during an upper GI endoscopy. The most common of these is called a fundic gland polyp and is associated with the use of PPIs. Larger tumors, however, have the potential to ulcerate and bleed, causing pain and symptoms like those of a peptic ulcer. Removal of large tumors that cause symptoms and that can obstruct the digestive process is normally recommended.

Stomach polyps come in a variety of sizes from small to large and may be of no harm or may be on their way to becoming cancerous, just as colon polyps may be. The dangerous polyps are those that derive from intestinal metaplasia (adenocarcinomas), those that derive from the stomach itself (gastric lymphoma), and those caused by a mutation in connective tissues (gastrointestinal stromal tumors, or GIST).

GULP!

A rare stomach disorder known as Ménétrier disease is characterized by enlarged gastric folds, often with polyps and ulcers, that dramatically increase the weight and size of the stomach. Ménétrier disease is associated with protein loss in the stool and a 15 percent increased risk of gastric cancer.

Diagnosing and Treating Polyps

Although many polyps and tumors are found incidentally during an endoscopy, if large enough they may be felt by a doctor during a physical examination. Tenderness in the abdominal area may be present as well, but a diagnosis is not usually made until other potential problems are ruled out, such as gastric ulcers, enlarged blood vessels, or cancer. Other forms of testing—most likely an upper GI endoscopy with a biopsy—need to be conducted. Sometimes an endoscopic ultrasound (EUS) is performed to locate the depth of the tumor, revealing its degree of invasion as well as to biopsy the growth.

The removal of small polyps is done during an endoscopy by snaring and cauterizing the growth. Unfortunately, larger polyps may require surgery, and if multiple polyps are found, part of the stomach may need to be removed. Some people have a genetic predisposition to polyps in the stomach, particularly those that are precancerous.

Cancerous Conditions

As one might suspect, *H. pylori* is the most common cause of stomach cancer worldwide. Because it is responsible for much of the inflammation and most peptic ulcers, changes in the stomach lining, including precancerous ones, are usually attributed to this infection. As in Barrett's esophagus, where the lining of the esophagus changes to stomach and then intestinal tissue, *H. pylori* can alter the gastric lining to resemble the small intestine. These types of conditions are fertile ground for the development of cancer.

 GI DIDN'T KNOW!

Stomach cancer is most prevalent in Asian countries, including Japan, China, Taiwan, and particularly Korea, where it is the most common type of cancer.

Other causes of gastric cancer certainly exist. People who have had stomach surgery or suffer from atrophic gastritis or pernicious anemia are at a higher risk. In addition, chemical dusts and fumes in the workplace have been linked to stomach cancer, and many researchers believe that cigarette smoking also increases your risk. Whether or not diet has an effect in gastric cancer development is debatable. Foods high in preservatives and those cooked over charcoal have been implicated as potential carcinogens. Interestingly, however, it appears that regions of the world where foods are typically preserved through drying, smoking, salting, and pickling seem to have higher rates of stomach cancer than other locales.

Detecting Gastric Cancer

If gastric cancer is detected early, it can most definitely be cured. Unfortunately, most cases are not diagnosed until much later when the cancer is advanced and becomes more difficult to treat. Gastric cancer can spread along the stomach wall into the small intestine and esophagus and also can find its way to the liver, pancreas, and colon. In women, the ovaries are often targeted and may result in Krukenberg tumors—metastasized malignancies originating from the stomach or breast—in each ovary, a difficult condition to treat. In part because of its potential to spread, survival rates for stomach cancer appear dismal, although it is not unheard of to keep the cancer at bay for some time.

Symptoms and Warnings

Like many types of gastrointestinal (GI) cancer, stomach cancer often presents no symptoms in its early stage. When symptoms finally emerge, they tend to be vague and usually ignored or attributed to other disorders such as dyspepsia. One early warning sign is a full feeling in the stomach after eating a small amount. Later symptoms include the following:

- Indigestion and heartburnlike sensations

- Pain or discomfort in the abdominal region

- Nausea and vomiting

- Diarrhea or constipation

- Bloating after meals

- Loss of appetite, often for meat

- Blood in vomit or stool

- Fatigue and weakness

- Weight loss

TUMMY TIP

If you have any family members with stomach cancer, it would be a good idea to be tested periodically, especially if you are over 50. Genetic susceptibility is a known factor, and having blood type A appears to increase your risk as well.

Because many of these symptoms are similar to those of numerous other GI disorders, your doctor will rule out as many other conditions as possible before suggesting the likelihood of gastric cancer.

Tests, Staging, and Treatment

Diagnosing gastric cancer is done with an upper GI endoscopy and biopsy so that stomach tissue can be examined for the presence of cancer cells. Blood work is also done and possibly an upper GI series with barium (see Chapter 4). Once a diagnosis of cancer is confirmed, tests such as a CT scan (see Chapter 4) and/or ultrasound will help to determine if and where any spread has taken place. These tests also help in staging the cancer, but until surgery has taken place and nearby lymph nodes and organs are tested, staging will not be complete.

Stomach cancer, as well as many other forms of cancer, is staged according to the TNM (tumors, nodes, and metastases) classification system. This type of staging provides a global standard for physicians to assist in treatment planning and prognosis. Not all tumors are classified this way (brain tumors are an exception), but in general, defining the extent of the cancer using the three TNM elements is an important aspect of cancer evaluation. (See esophageal cancer staging as an example in Chapter 6.)

GI DIDN'T KNOW!

A rare type of gastric cancer known as mucosa-associated lymphoid tissue (MALT) lymphoma can actually regress after treating *H. pylori* present with antibiotics.

Surgery is by far the most common treatment for gastric cancer, with the removal of the tumor or part of the stomach taking place. A complete gastrectomy—removal of the entire stomach—may be necessary, depending on the individual case. The esophagus would then be connected directly to the small intestine. Clearly, much healing time is necessary after gastric surgery, and intravenous feeding is the norm until the patient can ingest liquids and soft foods.

In addition to surgery, most patients usually undergo a combination of therapies including chemotherapy and radiation. Many clinical trials make use of biological therapy, also called immunotherapy, which helps your immune system destroy cancer cells by specifically targeting certain molecules involved with the disease as well as recover from some of the side effects of other treatments. Although stomach cancer is an extremely serious disease, new chemotherapy regimes have recently improved long-term survival rates in some patients, even in advanced cases. For example, a new drug called Gleevec has had excellent results in preventing the recurrence of GIST.

The Least You Need to Know

- Gastritis is an inflammation of the stomach lining and may or may not cause symptoms.
- Gastritis is easily treated with medication and a change in diet.
- Ulcer disease results from acute or chronic inflammation and erosion of the stomach or duodenal lining.
- Most gastritis and peptic ulcers are caused by either *H. pylori* bacteria infection, which is treated with antibiotics, or NSAIDs.
- Ulcers can bleed or perforate and become life-threatening if left untreated.
- Some people are more susceptible to stomach cancer, which is often caused by *H. pylori* and genetic factors.

Celiac Disease

In This Chapter

- Gluten and your health
- Symptoms and repercussions of celiac disease
- Confirming your condition and changing your diet

For centuries, wheat has been a staple of human existence. Agriculture-driven societies have thrived because of it, and many cultural traditions have been based on its consumption. What would Italian cooking be without pasta? Or Jewish heritage without matzo? For many, it's unthinkable to eat without wheat, but for a growing number of people, wheat—specifically the substance called gluten that it contains—can wreak havoc on their daily digestive health and jeopardize their future overall health as well.

We'll explore the digestive condition known as celiac disease in this chapter and take a look at how it is diagnosed and treated. We'll also learn who is at risk of developing it and what the symptoms may be when they arise. Like many other digestive disorders, celiac disease can often be confused with other gastrointestinal (GI) conditions. But with modern testing techniques and a growing awareness of its increasing existence, doctors are often able to detect celiac disease before irreparable damage occurs.

Celiac disease is one of the few digestive disorders that responds almost immediately to a change in diet. Once the disease is diagnosed, strict adherence to gluten-free eating keeps symptoms in check and allows the healing process to work in most cases. In some rare instances, however, dietary changes may not be enough. We'll look at such cases as well. We'll also discover the most current treatment and research being conducted on a disorder that is estimated to affect nearly two million Americans.

When Gluten Is the Enemy

Celiac disease, also called sprue or *gluten* sensitive enteropathy (GSE), occurs when your small intestine reacts negatively after digesting gluten in wheat and other types of grains, including barley and rye. Your immune system sees gluten as a foreign substance that it must attack. In the process, the small intestine becomes inflamed and damaged, causing problems with the absorption of nutrients, a situation that can ultimately lead to deficiency-related illnesses and even cancer.

DEFINITION

Gluten is a sticky protein found in wheat and other grains, and it is what gives wheat dough its elastic texture. Its name comes from the Latin word for glue.

Gluten itself is a combination of other proteins called gliadin and glutenin. In actuality, it is the gliadin protein that people with celiac disease cannot tolerate and that causes the immune system to go on the attack.

Allergy or Sensitivity?

Although an autoimmune disorder, celiac disease is not an allergy to wheat or gluten per se; instead, it is a type of intolerance or sensitivity. Although people with celiac disease produce antibodies, the "allergic" process is not the same. In typical allergies, antibodies attack or bind themselves to allergens and release chemicals that produce classic allergy symptoms such as itching, sneezing, or—in the case of food allergies—difficulty swallowing or breathing (see Chapter 17). For example, after eating food containing wheat, someone with a wheat allergy could experience hives, nausea, or even a life-threatening reaction called anaphylaxis, in which the entire body severely reacts to the allergen, potentially causing respiratory failure, low blood pressure, and death. The reaction is different with celiac disease.

GULP!

Don't confuse your wheat with your gluten. People with a wheat allergy are able to eat other grains that celiacs cannot. Celiac sufferers, on the other hand, must shun wheat, barley, and rye because they contain gluten.

Villi in Distress

The antibodies created by celiac sufferers, in an attempt to combat gluten, end up attacking the body itself, specifically the upper small intestine and its fingerlike, delicate projections called villi. Inflammatory cells called T-cells do even more damage. We met villi in Chapter 2 when we discussed the role of the small intestine as a digestive team player. These little projections are responsible for finishing the processing of chyme and absorbing nutrients from food into the bloodstream. Normal, healthy villi are quite perky and upright, able to do their job without a hitch. Unfortunately for those with celiac disease, the villi—after repeated inflammatory attacks—become plump and swollen, causing digestive distress. Eventually they lose their perkiness altogether and become flat and blunt, losing a lot of surface area, sort of like an old squashed shag carpet that's lost its characteristic poof. Once this happens, the villi's function is greatly impaired, and they are unable to absorb much of the nutrition we require. As a result, conditions related to specific nutritional deficiencies can arise as well as some rather distressing GI symptoms such as diarrhea and abdominal pain.

All in the Family

Celiac disease definitely runs in families. If a grandparent, parent, or sibling has the disease, there is a 10 percent chance that you may, too. The most current research shows that, in order to develop celiac disease, it is necessary to have at least one of the two identified genes associated with it, HLA-DQ2 or HLA-DQ8. Statistics bear this research out; more than 97 percent of celiac patients do indeed have one of these genes. Being genetically predisposed, however, does not mean you will definitely develop the disorder, but it does increase your chances and also makes you a carrier of the genes to your offspring. If you don't possess at least one of these genes, your chance of developing celiac disease is generally slim to none.

A Heritage Trail

Your ethnic heritage and background may be a factor in whether you carry the genes that put you at risk of becoming a celiac sufferer. Caucasians of Western European descent are most often affected. In fact, celiac disease is the most common genetic disease known in Europe, particularly in countries such as England, Ireland, Spain, and Italy. But recent studies have shown an increased prevalence in Eastern Europe, too, as well as in South America and northern Africa. People of Asian descent, however, appear to be largely unaffected. Estimated percentages in the United States have varied, but it is believed we are well on our way to matching those of Western Europe.

GI DIDN'T KNOW!

In Italy, about 1 in 250 people have celiac disease. Because of this high percentage, the government health system tests all adolescent and adult Italians who display even slight symptoms and has begun testing all children by the age of 6.

Increased Risk

Some people who are genetically predisposed to celiac disease may have an even greater risk of developing the disease than other predisposed individuals. The American Gastroenterological Association (AGA) has identified the following disorders that are sometimes associated with the disease and that warrant testing for celiac disease under certain circumstances:

* Iron-deficiency anemia

* Premature osteoporosis

* Adult osteoporosis that doesn't respond to treatment

* Type 1 diabetes

* Autoimmune thyroid disease

* Female reproductive disorders

* Liver disease

* Irritable bowel syndrome (IBS)

* Down syndrome

* *Turner syndrome*

* Epilepsy with no known cause

DEFINITION

Turner syndrome is a female genetic disorder caused by a missing or defective X chromosome, usually resulting in the failure of ovaries to develop. Girls may be short in stature, have hearing problems, and display a number of distinct physical traits such as abnormal nails and small lower jaws.

Symptoms of Celiac Disease

One of the frustrating aspects of celiac disease is that everyone is affected differently. Another is that often, particularly in adults, symptoms are nonexistent until later in life or until secondary disorders arise that might prompt investigation. An interesting British study actually showed that many people with undiagnosed celiac disease had quite a good quality of life. They were slender, fit, and free of the usual middle-age health problems associated with obesity, such as diabetes and heart disease, until suddenly, in their 50s and 60s, the long-term effects of celiac disease kicked in and they became quite seriously ill.

It is also possible for the disease to lie dormant for many years, only to be triggered by some type of life trauma such as pregnancy, childbirth, surgery, stress, or infection. Delayed onset may have something to do with whether or not you were breast-fed. Researchers believe that breast-feeding could somehow cause symptoms to develop later rather than sooner. It is also believed that starting to eat gluten-containing foods at a later childhood age rather than during early development could delay symptoms as well.

GULP!

If you are free of symptoms, it could be that the undamaged part of the small intestine is, for the present, still able to absorb enough nutrients. However, celiac disease progresses and leads to malnutrition as well as other conditions if left untreated.

Gastrointestinal Signs

At one time, there were three classic symptoms that physicians looked for when suspecting celiac disease: nocturnal diarrhea, weight loss, and abdominal pain. However, these no longer seem to hold true for the majority of sufferers. Instead, there is a huge array of possible symptoms, either GI or related to malabsorption, that could appear depending on the individual. Potential digestive-related symptoms include the following:

- Bloating

- Chronic indigestion

- Diarrhea

- Abdominal pain and cramping

- Pale, sticky, and fatty stool

- Constipation

- Mouth ulcers

- Lactose intolerance (see Chapter 17)

Many of these symptoms can also be attributed to IBS, Crohn's disease (CD), or stomach ulcers and would need to be evaluated in the context of other symptoms and diagnostic testing.

Signs of Malabsorption

Once villi are damaged and unable to absorb nutrients properly, other symptoms can occur that might indicate celiac disease. These symptoms include the following:

- **Weight loss and fatigue:** Because of inability to absorb carbohydrates and fats

- **Anemia:** From the malabsorption of iron, folic acid, or vitamin B_{12}

- **Osteoporosis:** From a lack of calcium and vitamin D

- **Abnormal blood coagulation:** Caused by a vitamin K deficiency and evident in a higher risk of bleeding or bruising

Irritability or depression can also be a sign of celiac disease, particularly in children, who may show stunted growth or what is referred to as "failure to thrive."

The Gluten Rash

Dermatitis herpetiformis (DH), often referred to as gluten rash, is also caused by gluten intolerance. It is not a symptom of celiac disease; rather, it is a separate disease that can occur alongside celiac disease or even in its absence. DH is characterized by an extremely itchy and burning rash manifesting in clusters of water blisters and small red bumps. Usually developing on the elbows and knees, the rash can also appear on the back, scalp, neck, and buttocks.

People who suffer from this often unbearable gluten rash usually do not have any digestive problems along with it, although the same intestinal damage seen with celiac disease may still occur. In fact, about 66 percent of DH sufferers show damage to the villi in the small intestine. Often hitting in the teenage years, DH is seen in all age groups and with people who have the same ethnic background commonly seen in celiac disease patients.

Getting a Diagnosis

Thanks to a growing recognition of celiac disease among the medical community and the public, getting a proper diagnosis may not take as long as it once did. It has been estimated that in the past, the unfortunate norm for Americans was an average of 10 years from the onset of symptoms to the diagnosis of celiac disease. Today, that span is greatly decreasing. Current diagnostic testing and a keen awareness on the part of gastroenterologists has made it easier to reach a definitive conclusion earlier rather than later.

Checking for Antibodies

The first line of inquiry is a full discussion with your doctor of any symptoms you may have as well as a thorough physical exam. Next a blood test checks for antibodies. In the past, only levels of antibodies to gluten such as antigliadin and antiendomysium, determined by an *immunoglobulin A (IgA)* test, were used. Currently, a blood test for antibodies to tissue transglutaminase (anti-tTG) is nearly 99 percent accurate in identifying celiac disease, although IgA results are still examined in the overall diagnosis.

DEFINITION

Immunoglobulin A (IgA) is a type of antibody produced in the nose, throat, lungs, and gut in response to what your body perceives are foreign substances you have breathed in or ingested. This antibody helps to prevent bronchitis, pneumonia, and infections of the digestive tract.

The Necessity of a Biopsy

Even though blood tests may be positive for celiac disease, guidelines recommend that further testing through biopsy confirm or negate the diagnosis. An upper endoscopy to obtain small pieces of tissue for examination also allows the gastroenterologist to take a good look at the inner surface of the small intestine to check for telltale signs of the disease. Often a scalloping of the folds in the lining can be seen or a "cracked mud" appearance may be detected on the surface. When the tissue samples are examined under a microscope, the pathologist looks to see if the villi are flattened, indicating damage and an inability to do their usual job of nutrient absorption.

If your doctor notes visual signs of DH, a biopsy of the skin instead of the small intestine will likely be done. In this case, the pathologist looks for signs of IgA deposits in the blisters or bumps. To be accurate, however, either a skin biopsy or small intestine biopsy needs to be done while you are still ingesting gluten. If you have been trying a gluten-free diet on your own, you need to inform your doctor, in which case you may be required to ingest gluten-containing foods for a period of time—called a gluten challenge—before a biopsy can be performed. Otherwise, false negatives may result, making it more difficult to obtain a definitive diagnosis.

Treatment and Follow-Up

The great news is that once you begin to follow a gluten-free diet, celiac disease can be cured in 99 percent of cases. In fact, within days you will begin to feel better, while any digestive symptoms you may have experienced will gradually disappear. Even the little villi will stand erect again and start to do their job. A dietician or nutritionist may be recommended for you, and your doctor will no doubt give you copious information about gluten-free foods and resources. It will be up to you to follow the drill. Complete healing may take three to six months, perhaps longer for elderly patients. But for the most part, if you stick to a careful eating plan, your troubles will be over.

GULP!

Unlike food allergies that you can sometimes outgrow, celiac disease requires a lifetime of gluten-free eating. Just because your symptoms have disappeared doesn't mean the disease has, too. Sometimes symptoms can come back with even greater force if you return to eating gluten.

Patients with a diagnosis of DH that does not respond to a gluten-free diet probably will require medication in the form of dapsone, an antibacterial drug originally used in the treatment of leprosy. Although DH and celiac disease are not bacteria driven, dapsone, which probably works by disrupting normal functioning of an inflammatory cell called a monocyte, does extremely well when prescribed for skin conditions such as DH and other autoimmune skin disorders. It may be necessary to stay on the drug for a number of years until the rash has been resolved. While you are taking dapsone, your doctor will perform periodic blood tests to check for anemia, a common side effect.

More Testing?

Unfortunately, although nothing more than a change in diet is generally required for the treatment of celiac disease, the only way your doctor really knows for sure that the diagnosis was correct and the disease has been put to rest is to conduct more tests. He or she needs to know whether the gluten-free diet has succeeded in reducing the number of antibodies and whether your small intestine has healed from the damage. This follow-up definitely requires blood work and possibly a repeat biopsy, particularly if symptoms persist. In the majority of cases, however, people who do not improve either are not following the diet (and saying they are) or are unknowingly ingesting foods containing gluten. Even small, hidden amounts can cause symptoms to continue. For this reason, working with a dietician may be helpful. Rarely, however, diet may not be the answer, and further treatment therapies may be necessary.

When Diet Is Not Enough

In an extremely small number of cases, people with celiac disease may not improve on a gluten-free diet despite vigilant adherence. When the immune system does not respond to diet changes, the case may be one of refractory sprue, a resistant form of the disease. In general, older people who have had celiac disease for a long time and have sustained severe damage to the small intestine are the primary candidates for developing this resistant form. In some instances, short-term use of steroids can help the disease respond to dietary changes. In other cases, particularly for those who are experiencing severe weight loss and chronic fatty-type diarrhea, immunosuppressive drugs and intravenous nutritional feeding may be necessary.

In about 75 percent of refractory sprue patients, there is a consistently high level of *lymphocytes* in the lining of the small intestine. The presence of these lymphocytes could indicate precancerous changes in the cells and eventually lymphoma or cancer of the small bowel. Refractory sprue may also result in a Crohn's-like disease of the small intestine called ulcerative jejunitis, named after the jejunum or middle portion of the small bowel where it occurs. This condition is often found during a small bowel capsule endoscopy that can explore the small intestine in greater detail and that is usually used to diagnose refractory sprue. Sometimes a colonoscopy is conducted as well to check for lymphocyte damage in the colon, a condition called microscopic colitis (see Chapter 9).

DEFINITION

Lymphocytes are a type of white blood cell in the immune system that play an integral role in the body's defenses against disease. The three major types of lymphocytes are T cells, B cells, and natural killer (NK) cells.

Living With Celiac Disease

Make no mistake, learning to eat gluten free is no easy task, but it can definitely be done. Once you begin to carefully examine many of the products you normally buy, you'll be amazed to discover that gluten can weasel its way into the most unlikely places. From condiments to soups to baked goods, gluten in its various forms can make an appearance where you least expect it. Once you know what to look for, however, you'll become quite the expert at sifting through the options and zeroing in on the stuff you'll want to buy and keep on hand.

Separating the Wheat from the Safe

Remember that gluten, not simply wheat, is what you need to avoid. There are other grains as well that you have to watch out for, each with its own type of gluten protein. They include the following:

- Wheat (gliadin)
- Spelt (gliadin)
- Triticale (gliadin)
- Kamut (gliadin)
- Rye (secalin)
- Barley (hordein)
- Oats (avenin)

Some people are able to tolerate oat gluten and products that contain it (such as oatmeal) after intestinal healing is well underway. Be sure to consult your dietician or doctor about how to reintroduce oats into your diet if you would like to do so. Remember that wheat includes farina, graham, semolina, durum, bulgur, and matzo—all off limits in any amount.

Picking Flours

At first glance, it may seem that virtually any type of food made with flour is not allowed on a gluten-free diet. There are, however, numerous other types of flours and meals that are perfectly safe and that are often used in baking and cooking. Here are some safe choices:

- Corn

- Rice

- Potato

- Quinoa

- Buckwheat

- Amaranth

- Soy and other beans

Many delicious gluten-free products, from breads to pasta to cookies, are made with these types of flours. Be sure to look for labels that read "gluten free" to be sure. When labeling is not clear, it is often best to avoid purchasing items until you are able to contact the manufacturer to be sure they are entirely gluten free and have not been subject to *cross-contamination*. The Food Allergen Labeling and Consumer Protection Act (FALCPA), which took effect in 2006, requires food labels to clearly identify wheat and other common food allergens in the list of ingredients. The U.S. Food and Drug Administration is currently developing and finalizing rules for the use of the term "gluten free" on all product labels, which will make it easier for shoppers to identify safe products.

DEFINITION

Cross-contamination occurs at manufacturing plants when the same machinery and tools process different ingredients. For example, wheat gluten could contaminate oats in a plant that makes both wheat cereal and oatmeal.

Hide and Seek

Because gluten can be present in unexpected places, it's extremely important to make a habit of reading labels. Food additives such as modified food starch, preservatives, and stabilizers made from wheat are often found in commercial products. Even lipsticks and mouthwash may contain these types of ingredients. Although many supermarkets are now carrying gluten-free products for your convenience, you may still want to visit your local health-food store from time to time for particularly unusual items. New gluten-free products appear every day, and you will find that living with celiac disease no longer means depriving yourself of your favorite things.

Many restaurants now boast gluten-free items on their menus, local bakeries often cater to gluten-free demands, and there is even a gluten-free beer you can buy!

The Future of Gluten Free

Much research is now ongoing in order to make life easier and more satisfying for those with celiac disease. Clinical trials are exploring the effectiveness of new medications and enzymes that could block the autoimmune reaction by digesting the gluten in a special way before it hits the small intestine. New wheat variants are being cultivated that gluten-free eaters may one day safely consume. As we learn more about this disease, more solutions for coping with it will emerge. In addition, if early screening becomes the norm, fewer people will be in danger of long-term complications to their digestive health and their overall quality of life.

The Least You Need to Know

- Celiac disease is an inherited condition in which ingested gluten—a protein in wheat, rye, and barley—cannot be tolerated.
- If left untreated, celiac disease damages the small intestine, creates nutrient malabsorption, and can lead to cancer.
- Symptoms do not always appear, even though damage to the digestive system may be present.
- Diagnosis involves blood tests and, in most cases, a biopsy of the small intestine or skin.
- Celiac disease is treated by eliminating all gluten from the diet, a lifetime requirement.
- Learning about safe food selection, substitutions, and hidden sources of gluten helps to manage the disease and allow for a satisfying, symptom-free life.

Lower GI Conditions and Diseases

Now it's time to explore the lower gastrointestinal system and the conditions and diseases that could affect it. From the lower small bowel through the colon and rectum, many diseases dwell in this area—Crohn's disease, ulcerative colitis, and irritable bowel syndrome to name a few. We hear more and more about these conditions, and they appear to be more prevalent every day. We'll take a look at why this may be the case, how you can get a proper diagnosis, and what treatments and medications seem to be the best for these debilitating diseases.

You'll also learn about colon polyps and colon cancer, topics that are often avoided or misunderstood. You'll never shun the dreaded colonoscopy again once you learn the vital importance of routine checkups. Other lower gastrointestinal conditions will be covered as well, including diverticulitis and appendicitis, so get ready to dive in and learn everything you need to know about the possible problems and solutions facing your lower gut.

Crohn's Disease and Ulcerative Colitis

In This Chapter

- Investigating inflammatory bowel disease
- Diagnosing and treating Crohn's disease
- Understanding ulcerative colitis

Crohn's disease (CD) and ulcerative colitis (UC) are the two main types of what physicians refer to as inflammatory bowel disease (IBD). Not to be confused with IBS, or irritable bowel syndrome (see Chapter 10), these conditions share a number of similar symptoms and treatments, and they are usually discussed together. However, Crohn's and UC have distinct differences, which we'll look at in detail in this chapter.

Although IBD definitely affects your quality of life, serious life-threatening complications do not often arise. Still, the severity of IBD is very real, and it must be treated as a chronic condition for the rest of your life. The goal of treatment is to put the disease into an inactive state called remission and to avoid painful flare-ups and severe complications such as severe malnutrition and bowel perforations. In most cases, a definitive diagnosis, followed by appropriate medications and occasionally dietary changes, resolves both mild and moderate symptoms. Surgery, in some instances, may be recommended or required.

Two Inflammatory Conditions

Inflammatory bowel disease, or IBD, is the term physicians use to encompass a group of inflammatory conditions of the digestive tract. CD and UC are the two main types of IBD, although other less common diseases fall under this category as well, including microscopic colitis, Behçet's syndrome, and chronic ischemic colitis (see Chapter 12). Because many of these diseases—particularly Crohn's and UC—have very similar symptoms and are sometimes difficult to diagnose early, doctors may refer to your IBD as *indeterminate colitis* (*ID*) until a more definitive diagnosis can be made.

DEFINITION

Indeterminate colitis (ID) is the diagnosis given when a patient has overlapping symptoms of both CD and UC. Eventually, most cases of ID are definitively diagnosed as Crohn's.

What's the Difference?

The primary differences between the two major types of IBD—CD and UC—involve the location and the nature of the inflammation. CD can affect any part of the digestive tract from beginning (mouth) to end (anus), but it is most often found in the colon and the terminal ileum, the lower part of the small intestine closest to the colon. This is why CD was once referred to as terminal ileitis. UC, on the other hand, is generally restricted to the colon and rectum. In addition, CD typically affects the entire bowel wall, whereas UC affects only the mucosa, the moist inner lining of the digestive tract. The issue of abdominal pain can also be a bit different, with pain being a more prominent symptom of CD overall, felt most often on the right-lower quadrant near the terminal ileum. Pain associated with UC is more often felt on the lower-left side.

Symptom Similarities

For the most part, both CD and UC display similar symptoms, including the following:

- Abdominal cramps and pain

- Bloody diarrhea

- An urgency to eliminate

- Loss of appetite

- Weight loss

- Anemia due to blood loss or vitamin B_{12} deficiency

In addition, other types of symptoms that are not digestive can appear with IBD, primarily resulting from the body's response to inflammation. The following are a few examples:

- Fever

- Fatigue

- Joint pain

- Eye swelling and redness

- Skin rashes

- Canker sores, called aphthous ulcers

Both conditions may remain in remission with only periodic acute flare-ups. But a chronic display of symptoms can also develop in either at any time before being diagnosed and treated.

Let's take a closer look at these two major types of IBD and discover the possible causes, potential complications, and the most current diagnostic techniques and treatment available for each.

What Is Crohn's Disease?

Crohn's disease, or CD, is an autoimmune disorder in which the body's immune system attacks the gastrointestinal (GI) tract. Exactly why it does so is not really known, but in essence, the immune system, either mistakenly or in an overactive defensive mode, deems bacteria and other substances in the tract to be foreign. Chronic inflammation is the result, typically with the symptoms mentioned previously, particularly cramping, pain, and diarrhea. Although any area of the digestive tract can be affected, inflammation tends to occur most often in those areas where there is a dense presence of immune cells such as the terminal ileum and rectum.

GI DIDN'T KNOW!

Lesniowski's disease? An American gastroenterologist, Burrill Bernard Crohn, described what we now refer to as Crohn's disease in 1932, but a Polish surgeon named Antoni Lesniowski was actually the first to report the condition in 1904.

The three main categories of Crohn's are named for the areas of the digestive tract where they most often occur.

Ileocolic Crohn's affects the last part of the small intestine (ileum) and usually the first part of the large intestine (colon). Ileocolic Crohn's is the finding in 50 percent of cases.

Crohn's ileitis affects only the ileum (intestine) and makes up 30 percent of cases.

Crohn's colitis affects only the large intestine and is the finding in 20 percent of cases. This last type, primarily affecting the colon, is most often confused with UC and may result in a diagnosis of indeterminate colitis until more revealing evidence is found.

Who Is at Risk?

More and more evidence has shown that CD has a clear genetic link. In fact, if you have a sibling with CD, you are 30 times more likely to develop CD than the average person. The parent-to-child link is also a relatively strong one. Crohn's does not seem to differentiate between the sexes, with both men and women affected equally. Age, however, does appear to play a role, with most cases being diagnosed in patients during their late teens or between 20 and 30 years of age. Middle-age occurrence is less common, but an increase in people diagnosed with CD between 50 and 70 years of age has been noted. On occasion young children can develop CD, which is often detected when the normal growth process seems to be stunted. For reasons unknown, children born in the winter are more likely to develop CD than those born during other seasons of the year.

GULP!

Smoking not only increases the risk of developing CD, but can coax it out of remission and cause repeated flare-ups. Smoking can also reduce the effectiveness of CD medications.

Ethnic background plays a part in the prevalence of CD as well. People of Jewish heritage tend to be more likely to develop the disease, while African Americans exhibit a lower-than-average occurrence. Northern European and North American industrialized countries tend to see more cases of Crohn's than underdeveloped countries. This fact has led some researchers to believe that our modern diet may play a role in CD's development. Although a definitive link with diet has not yet been determined, there is a clear link with smoking, with smokers three times more likely to develop CD. There also appears to be a strong association between the use of oral contraceptives for birth control, begun in the 1960s, and a dramatic increase in the occurrence of CD.

Cause or Effect?

Until recently, it was thought that CD was a classic type of autoimmune disease like rheumatoid arthritis, in which an overzealous immune system goes on the attack, causing inflammation. However, current genetic research suggests that an underactive immune system may actually be at work. This impaired immune reaction would explain, at least in part, why the colon is often involved. The immune system's inability to interact correctly with the colon and colonic bacteria could result in chronic inflammation involving the bacteria themselves as well as the immune response. Understanding this flawed interaction could change the way that CD is viewed and treated in the future, particularly in the development of appropriate medications. This knowledge could also create a larger role for the introduction of healthy bacteria (called probiotics) in treating the disease.

Complications of Crohn's

Because the inflammation that occurs in patients with CD can span the entire depth of the intestinal wall, specific complications can arise that are not seen in UC, where only the inner lining is usually inflamed. These complications can create mechanical problems within the digestive tract resulting in blockage, bleeding, and pain, among other symptoms.

Intestinal Blockage

The most common complication of CD is blockage within the intestine. Blockage occurs when chronic inflammation, swelling, and scarring cause the walls to thicken, resulting in a smaller passageway for digested food to pass. If thickening is severe, the passageway can actually close and a blockage can occur. At this point the intestinal contents back up, resulting in constipation, vomiting, bloating, and intense pain.

GI DIDN'T KNOW!

Most intestinal food obstructions occur either in the middle of the night or just before lunch (the most common fasting states) when the stomach grumbles and opens wide, releasing large pieces of fiber (as well as swallowed chewing gum!) that can plug up the intestine.

Although rare in CD because of the increased thickness of the intestinal wall, a severe bowel obstruction could result in an intestinal wall perforation. This hole in the intestine could allow intestinal contents to enter the abdomen and result in a severe, life-threatening infection. Normally, however, partial and full obstructions are remedied by removing a buildup of fluid through a tube or reducing inflammation with medications so that the food mass (usually of high fiber) can pass naturally by itself. Cases that do not respond to anti-inflammatory drugs and other methods might require eventual surgery.

Fistulas and Abscesses

About one third of patients with CD develop what are called *fistulas*. Fistulas occur when a sore or ulcer resulting from chronic inflammation in the intestine erodes through the intestinal wall and forms a tunnel between the intestine and another organ or even to the surface of the body. Although areas around the rectum and anus are often involved, fistulas can occur anywhere along the intestinal tract.

DEFINITION

Fistulas or **fistulae** are abnormal connections or passageways between two organs or vessels that do not normally connect.

Fistulas can be distressing and painful. Examples include fistulas from the colon to the vagina, causing stool to leak from the vagina, or from the bowel directly to the skin, where stool also leaks. A fistula from the bowel to the bladder might cause flatus to pass in the urine as well as have recurrent bladder infections. These are disturbing events, to say the least.

Pain from fistulas can be a real concern, especially when infection is present. If the infection has nowhere to drain, it may be walled off in an abscess, an infected cavity that can be life threatening. Sometimes infected fistulas need to be surgically drained by an experienced surgeon or radiologist. Similarly, anal abscesses that become fistulas are also sometimes seen in Crohn's sufferers. Often mistaken for hemorrhoids by the patient, these fistulas cause increased pain over a short time and do not respond to over-the-counter hemorrhoid treatments. Medical examination is necessary. In most cases, surgical drainage of the abscess is required to prevent a fistula from forming (connecting the rectum to the skin) as well as a serious systemic infection. Abscesses are drained using a computed tomography (CT) scan or ultrasound for guidance.

Malnutrition and More

Complications that go beyond mechanical problems can be common among CD sufferers. You may have nutritional complications because of malabsorption or because eating causes discomfort. In particular, the small intestine's ileum, where most of our vitamin B_{12} is absorbed may be impaired, resulting in anemia. Advanced disease in the small intestine can make the body unable to absorb carbohydrates and fats properly as well, causing other nutritional deficiencies and weight loss. Further complications involving other organ systems can result if Crohn's is left untreated, including osteoporosis (thinning of the bones), eye inflammations (uveitis and episcleritis), arthritis (spondyloarthropathy), disturbing areas of necrotic skin, and severe skin blistering.

Up to 15 percent of Crohn's patients also develop neurological complications including seizures, stroke, headache, and depression. CD also increases the risk of cancer in the area where inflammation is present. Those whose small bowel is affected are more prone to small intestinal cancer, while patients with Crohn's colitis are at greater risk of developing colon cancer. The risk is up to 10 percent greater if the disease remains unchecked.

Diagnosing Crohn's Disease

Diagnosis of CD sometimes can be delayed by an average of five years, partly because of the few or vague symptoms that may show early in the disease. Often other less severe conditions such as IBS are assumed to be the cause of digestive distress. Frustrated sufferers have been known to try any number of remedies, including diet changes and stress relief, on their own. Persistent flare-ups and increasing severity of symptoms when they occur, however, normally indicate that something more is at work and that some form of IBD, often Crohn's, is a real possibility.

GI DIDN'T KNOW!

When overall inflammation from CD is particularly severe, symptoms can mimic those of appendicitis or inflammation of the appendix. A CT scan, however, finds the difference. Sometimes even experienced radiologists and pathologists miss the diagnosis though.

Fortunately, specific symptoms related to the location of inflammation could be key to discovering Crohn's sooner than later—something an experienced and knowledgeable gastroenterologist would recognize. For instance, bloody diarrhea could indicate an inflamed colon, while severe pain and bloating might suggest the formation of a partial blockage through thickening. Similarly, severe anal pain and discharge could indicate IBD affecting the rectum, and the passing of gas or air through the urethra might suggest a fistula to the bladder. These types of symptoms, especially when accompanied by a collection of inflammatory signs in the body, should definitely raise a red flag to the trained eye and start you on the path to a proper diagnosis.

Taking a Close Look

A colonoscopy is by far the best way to check for CD affecting the colon and terminal ileum. Patchy inflammation, with some areas of the colon appearing normal, is a good indicator. In some patients the doctor may be able to see the terminal ileum, but the remaining small bowel cannot be viewed with the colonoscopy. In these instances, when upper intestinal areas are suspected of being affected, an upper endoscopy may be performed with the possibility of a small bowel capsule endoscopy as well. When disease in the anus is suspected, a colorectal surgeon may be called in to perform an examination while the patient is under anesthesia.

Other examinations such as a special MRI that detects inflammation of the small intestine or a capsule endoscopy might be helpful in diagnosing CD as well. These types of tests have more or less replaced the older barium x-ray tests that used to be routine, reducing the amount of radiation patients receive. When fistulas or abscesses are suspected, however, the CT scan may be used as a possible method of diagnosis, further investigation, or in some cases actual treatment.

During the colonoscopy (or upper endoscopy), your gastroenterologist may collect tissue samples to be examined under a microscope. The pathologist then looks for signs of chronic inflammation such as an increase in chronic inflammatory cells (lymphocytes), changes in *Paneth cells*, and other abnormalities.

> **DEFINITION**
>
> **Paneth cells** are found in the intestinal tract and contribute to its maintenance by secreting enzymes when exposed to bacteria or bacterial antigens. These enzymes are thought to help defend against microbes.

Blood and Fecal Tests

Your doctor will also conduct a complete blood count (CBC) to reveal signs of anemia from blood loss or vitamin B_{12} deficiency. As mentioned before, low levels of B_{12} are common, especially when the ileum is involved since it is in this small bowel area where vitamin B_{12} is absorbed. Measurements of C-reactive protein (CRP) and erythrocyte sedimentation rate (ESR) can help determine the degree of inflammation. Sometimes a test for antibodies (IBD-7) may also help in both diagnosis and planning for the disease.

You may have fecal tests. Testing feces for blood, other signs of infection, and the presence of certain proteins associated with inflammation may help to eliminate other possible causes of your symptoms while helping to confirm a diagnosis of CD.

Sometimes a battery of tests that eliminates other causes helps your doctor reach a final diagnosis. The more information gained from diagnostic testing, the quicker your disease can be identified and treatment can begin.

Treating Crohn's Disease

Because there is no cure for CD, the primary goals are to get the disease under control and then keep it in remission for as long as possible. In order for the intestinal tract to heal and symptoms such as diarrhea and abdominal pain to subside, Crohn's needs to be addressed head on with medication. A number of new drugs have been developed recently that are proving to be successful in treating CD. Everyone is unique, and many drugs affect people differently, so your doctor will want to customize your medication and carefully monitor the progress it is making (or not making) in improving your condition.

Drug Therapy

The most common types of drugs used to treat CD are as follows:

- *Aminosalicylates:* These drugs contain mesalamine, a substance that helps control inflammation. Also known as 5-ASA drugs, sulfasalazine was once the most commonly used of this type, but others have now replaced it. New forms of 5-ASA drugs include suppositories and enemas that deliver the highest concentration of medicine at the site of the disease. Side effects are rare, but kidney problems as well as reduced male fertility have occurred. In mild cases of Crohn's, this drug may be enough to control the disease and maintain remission.

- *Corticosteriods:* This group includes steroids such as prednisone and is also anti-inflammatory in nature. They are normally prescribed only for the short term and are not recommended for maintenance. Side effects can be disagreeable (weight gain, personality changes, and acne), and patients are more susceptible to infection because the drugs suppress the immune system. For Crohn's that affects the ileum and/or the first upper part of the colon, a newer type of steroid called Entocort (budesonide) actually targets only the intestine and has been successful in greatly reducing side effects.

- *Immunomodulators:* These drugs also suppress the immune system, and doctors try them when the disease has become steroid dependent or when frequent flare-ups cannot be controlled by other drugs. Also called anti-metabolites, they include such drugs as 6-mercaptopurine, azathioprine, and methotrexate. However, liver and blood counts must be carefully monitored, and pancreatitis can sometimes occur. These drugs may cause side effects of nausea, vomiting, and diarrhea. These medicines sometimes take months to "kick in," so are best for maintaining someone who is already in remission from other medications.

- *Anti-TNF (tumor necrosis factor):* Technically considered a type of biologic therapy, drugs such as Humira, Cimzia, and Remicade (infliximab) may be used to treat moderate to severe cases, particularly when other drugs have not been effective. This class of medication works by blocking certain proteins that intensify inflammation in Crohn's.

TUMMY TIP

Speak to your doctor about any concerns you have about drug therapies, their side effects, and precautions. Anti-TNF drugs, as well as those that suppress the immune system, have been associated with severe infections and even lymphoma. Your doctor can help you weigh the pros and cons of your individual therapy versus the risk of ongoing severe disease.

- *Antibiotics:* These help heal fistulas and abscesses. Bacterial growth in the small intestine caused by stricture, fistulas, abscesses, or prior surgery may be treated with antibiotics as well. Either Cipro (ciprofloxacin) or Flagyl (metronidazole) or a combination of both are used, primarily when Crohn's is in an active stage, but they can also be helpful as part of long-term therapy. They are particularly effective when the colon is involved.

Nutrition and Diet

When treatment begins, depending on the severity of your disease and the length of time it has been active, malnutrition may be an issue. You may need a nutritional assessment to determine whether you are absorbing enough calories, vitamins, and minerals. Some patients may need to receive nutritional support, normally with a nutrient-rich liquid supplement delivered directly to the stomach or small bowel through a feeding tube down the nose or sometimes through a surgically created opening in the abdomen.

If the disease is active, doctors sometimes recommend what is called a "low-residue diet" (see Chapter 17). This diet often helps those whose Crohn's has specifically resulted in a thickening of the ileum from inflammation. Essentially a low-fiber diet, a low-residue diet may prevent potential blockages and alleviate gas, bloating, and pain while the intestine heals from swelling. Low-residue diets are also helpful to younger patients.

Studies are currently exploring ways in which diet and/or nutritional supplements can help recovery during initial treatment. Possible developments include the use of omega-3 fatty acids found in fish or flaxseed oil to reduce inflammation; probiotics to restore good intestinal flora; and vitamins and minerals such as calcium, selenium, and folic acid for healing.

Surgical Solutions

In some instances, surgery may be required to treat CD. Surgery is not the first choice of treatment and is used only in specific cases. This is because after surgery the disease eventually returns, usually at the site of the surgery. Any benefits are definitely temporary. Still, your doctor may recommend removing the diseased segment of the intestine and rejoining the healthy ends through a resection if your situation particularly warrants surgery. Such a case might be when medication does not work well, if there is a hole in the intestinal wall, if you experience excessive bleeding, or if a severe obstruction is present.

GULP!

The return of CD after surgery is generally predicted as a rule of three: one third will have mild CD, one third will still require medication, and one third will require further surgery.

A surgical procedure known as strictureplasty is more commonly performed for CD. This surgery widens a narrowed section of the intestine so that contents can move more freely through the digestive tract. Surgery may also be used to close fistulas and drain abscesses. Still, medication is an integral part of ongoing treatment, even after surgery, to avoid recurrence of the disease and will no doubt become an integral part of a lifelong maintenance plan.

Maintaining Remission

Once CD is in remission, you and your doctor want to keep it that way. Learning to prevent relapse is part of ongoing treatment, and there are a number of things you can do that will maximize your chances of keeping CD flare-ups at bay.

Medication Is Key

Even if you are feeling much better, you must continue to take medication that your doctor prescribes. Too often, patients become lax about pill taking only to have a sometimes horrific relapse occur. Remember, it is easier to maintain remission than to start it, so don't take any chances in this regard. If certain drugs are causing unpleasant side effects, speak with your doctor so you can develop an appropriate maintenance drug therapy plan that is best for you and one that you are more likely to stick with in the long term.

Be aware that many over-the-counter pain relievers can cause ulcerations in the intestinal tract and prompt a relapse. Aspirin, even coated tablets, as well as nonsteroidal anti-inflammatory drugs (NSAIDs) such as ibuprofen could be aggravating to your condition. Even the newer Cox-2 inhibitors such as Celebrex may need to be off limits. Inform your gastroenterologist if you are prescribed antibiotics by another physician for minor infections. Some patients have experienced flare-ups after antibiotic use or any other GI upset, so be sure to bring your doctor into the loop so he or she can, when appropriate, make recommendations for alternative types of antibiotics that are less likely to cause trouble.

Lifestyle and Diet

If you are a smoker, the most important lifestyle change you can make is to quit. Not only will smoking increase your chances of relapse, it will likely—especially after surgery—cause an increase in the severity of the disease. Try to become more physically active as well. Exercise contributes to healthy digestion, increases a low appetite, and improves your overall physical, mental, and emotional health. Even light exercise can be a great stress reliever.

Surprisingly, there is no evidence that your dietary history plays a role in the development of your CD. However, diet can certainly make a difference in reducing symptoms and promoting healing. There is no specific diet recommended during maintenance, and what works for some individuals may not be appropriate for others. For this reason, you should keep a food diary to alert you if specific types of foods cause discomfort and hint at a potential flare-up.

Some people find that dairy products increase their symptoms, especially immediately following an inflammatory episode. Others find that high-fiber foods create uncomfortable gas and bloating. Before you make any drastic changes to your diet, however, you must be sure you are getting enough calories and nutrition. Showing your food diary to a dietician will assist you both in developing an individual diet plan that fits your nutritional requirements, particularly if you are excluding certain foods.

Finally, depending on the extent and location of the disease, supplemental vitamins and minerals may be recommended during your maintenance. If the ileum has been damaged, vitamin B_{12} injections may be necessary. Iron supplements may be required, especially if chronic blood loss is an issue. In addition, some medications—such as the 5-ASA types—interfere with the absorption of folate (a B vitamin), so your doctor may recommend that you take folic acid supplements. Because osteoporosis is a real danger for Crohn's patients, calcium supplementation, along with vitamin D, may be recommended as well. These supplements are especially important if you are not consuming dairy products.

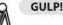

> **GULP!**
>
> Recent evidence suggests that folic acid supplementation may actually fuel the progression of colon cancer if precancerous conditions exist. Be sure to speak with your doctor about any nutritional supplements you take.

What Is Ulcerative Colitis?

In many ways, ulcerative colitis, or UC, is similar to Crohn's, as both are types of IBD. But, as noted earlier, UC is limited to the colon and rectal areas of the digestive tract, and the chronic inflammation that occurs does not, in most cases, extend beyond the depth of the inner lining of the intestine. In this way, UC would appear to be easier to diagnose. Unfortunately, many cases of CD affect the colon as well, so superficially, upon first inspection, many symptoms and characteristics are quite similar. (See the section on symptom similarities earlier in this chapter.)

Patterns of Inflammation

One of the most important differences in the appearance of the colon lining is that the patchiness of inflammation—often a hallmark of CD—is not seen in UC. Instead, the pattern of inflammation is more uniform, generally beginning at the rectum and encroaching continuously up through the colon to its uppermost area, the cecum, which connects to the ileum of the small intestine. For this reason, UC is usually categorized by the extent of the colon—from beginning to end—that is involved. These classifications have important implications when treatment, particularly with enemas, begins. The classifications by location are as follows:

- **Proctitis:** Limited to the rectum.

- **Proctosigmoiditis:** Involving the rectum and the sigmoid colon.

- **Left-sided colitis:** Involving the rectum and the sigmoid and descending colons.

- **Pancolitis:** Involving the rectum and the sigmoid, descending, and areas near the transverse colons. Pancolitis can be inflammation from rectum to transverse colon, or from rectum to cecum. Inflammation spreads beyond the *splenic flexure.*

DEFINITION

The **splenic flexure,** also called the left colic flexure, is a sharp bend between the transverse and descending colon, near where the spleen is located.

Pancolitis is often called extensive colitis because it is beyond the reach of enemas, having passed the splenic flexure. UC cases that do not reach this critical juncture are referred to as limited or distal colitis.

Classification of Severity

Inflammation associated with UC typically causes ulcers or open sores in the rectum and colon that may bleed and produce pus. This inflammation causes the colon to empty frequently, with constant bouts of diarrhea that are often bloody. The extent of the severity of UC and its progression is often categorized by the number of daily stools the patient experiences as well as other pertinent symptoms. These categories are as follows:

- **Mild:** Fewer than four stools, not necessarily bloody, with mild abdominal pain or cramping

- **Moderate:** More than four stools, not necessarily bloody, with moderate pain, possible anemia, and low-grade fever

- **Severe:** More than six bloody stools, anemia, fever, and rapid heartbeat

- **Fulminant:** More than 10 stools, continuous bleeding, abdominal tenderness and distension, and evidence of toxicity

When UC has progressed beyond the severe stage, there is a possibility that damage has gone deeper than the mucosal layer of the colon. As a consequence, billions of bacteria could enter the bloodstream, causing a systemic infection. Perforation of the colon could occur as well, leading to life-threatening circumstances. If motility, the contraction of intestinal muscles and movement of colon contents, is impaired and intense inflammation is present, *toxic megacolon* and death could result.

DEFINITION

Toxic megacolon is a life-threatening complication of UC and other intestinal conditions. It is characterized by an extremely dilated colon and abdominal bloating, with the possibility of bacteria flooding the bloodstream as well as septic shock leading to organ failure.

Complications and Risks

Because UC, like CD, is inflammatory in nature, many of the other organ system symptoms and complications related to Crohn's hold true for UC as well. Arthritic joint pain, eye and skin inflammation, sclerosing cholangitis (a chronic liver disease caused by inflammation and scarring), and clubbing are a few of the similarities. Because the small intestine, particularly the ileum, is not normally involved in UC, malabsorption of nutrients resulting in malnutrition is not as much of a concern as it is with Crohn's sufferers. Anemia, however, can be common from blood loss, and dehydration can be a real possibility when diarrhea is frequent.

Like CD, UC is generally considered to be an autoimmune disease in which the immune system goes on the attack resulting in inflammation. But whether it is the result of an overreaction or an abnormal or even underreaction of the system is currently under debate, as noted with CD. Also like Crohn's, diet and stress do not cause the disease but are likely to have an effect on an active episode and add to or alleviate some symptoms.

GI DIDN'T KNOW!

Remarkably, unlike with CD, smoking actually has some kind of positive effect on UC. Not only is UC less prevalent among smokers, it appears that smoking cessation can actually trigger a flare-up in those smokers who have UC. Although clearly not an excuse to smoke, patients with UC who are considering quitting should consult their doctor in order to minimize the chance of relapse.

In determining who may be at risk for developing UC, genetics again play a role as in CD. Having a close relative with UC increases your chances, and as with CD, age and ethnicity are a factor. Younger people (up to the age of 25) are more likely to get UC than older ones, although a spike in occurrences after age 50 is also seen. Northern European descendants, particularly of Jewish heritage, are more prone than others to both CD and UC. Males, however, seem to have a slight advantage, as they are a bit less likely than females to suffer from UC, unlike the 50-50 split seen with CD. In addition, having had an appendectomy appears to provide protection against UC for reasons that remain unclear.

Diagnosing and Treating Ulcerative Colitis

As with CD, initial testing involves blood work to reveal signs of anemia, inflammation, and possibly antibodies. Fecal tests help eliminate other possible causes of symptoms and check for bowel infections, which are typical in UC sufferers. However, the main diagnostic test is a colonoscopy with biopsy in order to make a definitive evaluation, although in mild cases a flexible sigmoidoscopy may be sufficient.

Drug Treatment

Once there is a diagnosis of UC and the extent and severity of the disease are known, your treatment begins with drug therapy. The medicines are the same ones used to treat CD, as shown in the following list. (See the section on Crohn's disease earlier in this chapter for further descriptions.)

- Aminosalicylates
- Corticosteriods
- Immunomodulators
- Anti-TNF (tumor necrosis factor)

As with CD, your doctor may prescribe a number of these drugs in combination to get your UC under control. Some may be used in pill form or as enemas to heal inflammation. Enemas have the benefit of being able to deliver a high concentration of drugs to the rectum where the inflammation starts and from where most symptoms emanate. In addition, other drugs may assist in reducing symptoms while the colon is healing. They may include the following:

- Antidiarrheals
- Pain relievers
- Iron supplements
- Nicotine patches

GULP!

Antidiarrheals and medicines such as loperamide (Immodium) to stop diarrhea must be used cautiously and under a doctor's supervision, as they can increase the chances of developing toxic megacolon in UC sufferers.

Surgical Treatment

In many cases, surgery can actually be curative for UC, unlike CD. Between 25 and 40 percent of people with UC eventually have surgery, either because of emergencies such as perforations of the colon, extensive bleeding, and toxic megacolon or because their chronic condition cannot be controlled adequately by medicine, although newer and more effective drugs such as Remicade may already be reducing these numbers.

When surgery is recommended, the procedure most often performed is the proctocolectomy—removal of the colon and rectum. In the past, after this surgery you would wear a small bag, called an ileostomy, over an opening in your abdomen to collect stool. But a procedure called ileoanal anastomosis eliminates the need to wear a bag. Instead, your doctor constructs a pouch from the end of your small intestine—referred to as a J pouch—that is then attached directly to the anus. Usually performed in two stages about two months apart, this procedure allows you to eliminate waste normally, although you may have more frequent bowel movements that are soft or watery because you no longer have a colon to absorb water.

Occasionally, some patients develop pouchitis, in which the created internal pouch becomes inflamed, although antibiotics normally reduce danger of infection. Those with sclerosing cholangitis, however, are at higher risk of developing pouchitis. Of greater concern for the majority of patients is the possibility of pouch failure, which necessitates the permanent use of an ileostomy outside the body to collect waste. For younger women, there may also be a decrease in fertility following this type of surgery.

Although surgery for UC, particularly the proctocolectomy, may seem emotionally trying, most patients find afterward that they are able to lead a better quality of life than when their UC was active. Support from family and friends, as well as local chapters of the Crohn's and Colitis Foundation of America (see the list of resources in Appendix B) where you can find *ostomates*, can help to relieve postsurgery fears and help with making lifestyle changes.

DEFINITION

Ostomates are people who live with ileostomies and who can help others understand how it affects a patient's lifestyle.

Guarding Against Colon Cancer

All patients with IBD that affects the colon, particularly those with severe UC or who develop sclerosing cholangitis, are at a high risk of developing colon cancer. The risk is as much as 10 times higher, especially after many years of the disease. Because of this increased possibility, it is important to have follow-up colonoscopies and biopsies to check for precancerous changes called dysplasia. It is generally recommended that screening, often called surveillance, take place within eight years of the initial disease activity, although depending on your circumstances your doctor may recommend earlier follow-ups. Precancerous changes in the colon can range from low to high, and when a high-grade level of dysplasia is found, a proctocolectomy is usually recommended.

The Least You Need to Know

- Crohn's disease (CD) and ulcerative colitis (UC) are the two main types of inflammatory bowel disease (IBD).
- Both CD and UC are considered to be autoimmune diseases in which the immune system attacks the digestive tract and causes inflammation.
- CD can occur anywhere from the mouth to the anus but is usually found in the small bowel ileum and the colon.
- UC is always limited to the colon and rectum and does not normally penetrate the inner intestinal lining.
- A number of drug therapies have been found to be successful at treating both CD and UC.
- Surgery is not usually recommended but may be necessary for Crohn's, while it can be curative for UC.

Irritable Bowel Syndrome

Chapter 10

In This Chapter

- What exactly is irritable bowel syndrome?
- The quest for a proper diagnosis
- The best treatment for you

The most common reason that people seek medical attention from a gastroenterologist may, in fact, be due to a condition known as irritable bowel syndrome (IBS). Estimated to affect up to 20 percent of the population—primarily women—this disorder, which involves the large intestine or colon, can dramatically alter the quality of a person's life. Although only a small number of people with IBS have severe symptoms and it does not cause any permanent damage to the colon, IBS can disrupt everyday activities with unpredictable, varied, and annoying digestive problems.

Once considered to be a purely psychosomatic phenomenon and dismissed as a woman's disease of stress, IBS has become the focus of much new research to get to the root of its causes and to develop appropriate therapies to treat it. Although there is no cure for IBS, there are many new ways to keep it under control, and we'll explore those options in this chapter.

We'll also closely examine the different ways that IBS can present itself because, very often, the symptoms for one person are quite different from those for another. We'll be revisiting the brain-belly connection as well because this appears to play a vital and interesting role in the way that IBS operates. Finally, we'll look at the role that diet and medication play in relieving uncomfortable symptoms and reducing their frequency so that IBS sufferers can lead a less stressful and more active, normal lifestyle.

What Is Irritable Bowel Syndrome?

To define exactly what IBS is and to understand the mechanisms at work behind it, let's first identify what IBS is *not*. Fortunately, unlike more serious intestinal diseases such as ulcerative colitis and Crohn's disease (CD), IBS does not cause inflammation or changes in bowel tissue such as ulcers or fistulas, nor does it increase your risk of developing colon cancer. It is not an infectious disease, an autoimmune disease, a food allergy or intolerance, or a form of inflammatory bowel disease (IBD). It does, however, tend to mimic many of these types of diseases and conditions so that it is often necessary to exclude them from the list of possibilities before a proper diagnosis can be made.

GI DIDN'T KNOW!

The term "irritable bowel syndrome" was first coined in an article appearing in the *American Journal of Gastroenterology* in 1967. Prior to that, it was referred to by many names, including colitis, mucous colitis, spastic colon, and spastic bowel.

The following is a list of other conditions that have symptoms similar to those of IBS. These conditions are sometimes mistakenly diagnosed prior to a thorough examination.

- Gynecological disorders, especially endometriosis
- Chronic digestive disorders involving poor diet, drugs, or bacteria
- Ischemia or poor blood flow to the intestines
- Cancer (ovarian or colon)
- Thyroid problems
- Celiac disease

Categorizing Symptoms

The symptoms of IBS can be numerous and quite different from person to person. However, there are some specific ones that are most often experienced and that assist physicians in categorizing the variations of IBS that are most often seen. These somewhat common symptoms include the following:

- Abdominal pain or cramping

- Bloating and gas

- Changes in bowel habits with diarrhea

- Changes in bowel habits with constipation

- *Tenesmus*

- Mucus in the stool

DEFINITION

Tenesmus is an uncomfortable sensation of needing to pass stool, usually with little result, or a feeling of incomplete emptying after a bowel movement.

In addition, up to 50 percent of patients may also suffer from occasional nausea, vomiting, and heartburn from functional dyspepsia or indigestion. Patients may experience any or all of the preceding symptoms, even during the course of one day, which is why IBS can be so tricky to diagnose.

TUMMY TIP

Certain symptoms send up a red flag that you are *not* suffering from IBS but should seek immediate medical attention to determine their potentially serious cause. They include bloody diarrhea, nocturnal urgency, and weight loss.

Part of formally defining IBS is that the symptoms—whatever they may be—are chronic. Patients should also experience some relief from these symptoms after a bowel movement. Still, despite the usual overlap of symptoms that can occur, IBS is normally technically categorized within the medical community according to its most prevalent symptom, as follows:

- IBS-D: When diarrhea is predominant

- IBS-C: When constipation is predominant

- IBS-A: When pain is predominant

A further classification, known as IBS-PI, is also sometimes used and stands for "post-infectious IBS." This is when the condition is believed to have a sudden, acute onset following an infectious illness, such as one caused by a virus or parasite in which fever, vomiting, or diarrhea was present.

Because many patients experience both diarrhea and constipation equally, they are sometimes included in the category of IBS-A or in another category referred to as IBS-M or "mixed." Keep in mind that these classifications—devised by the Rome Foundation, a group of international physicians who help to better understand and diagnose functional conditions such as IBS—are often revised and reviewed, and your doctor may not always refer to your condition in these terms. A good gastroenterologist who has extensive knowledge and experience with IBS will not pigeonhole your condition or be limited by these criteria in diagnosing and treating your illness.

Who Gets Irritable Bowel Syndrome?

IBS can develop at any age, but most cases are diagnosed in people between the ages of 15 and 40. Twice as many women as men are IBS sufferers, which has led researchers to suspect that female reproductive hormones may play a part, particularly because much of the pain and other symptoms women often experience occur during menstrual periods. There seems also to be a correlation between victims of physical and sexual abuse and those who develop IBS, which may be another reason why it is more common in women.

If a close family member, such as a parent or sibling, has IBS, it is somewhat more likely that you will also experience IBS symptoms. This may or may not be connected to a genetic factor, but it could point to a shared family environment, usually one that is detrimental in nature. Current research is exploring this possibility.

What Causes Irritable Bowel Syndrome?

Understanding the mechanics behind IBS helps to explain its possible causes. Although there is no one cause that is currently agreed upon, many believe that it involves an electrical system that has gone haywire within our personal plumbing system, a phenomenon we first visited in Chapter 1.

Mixed Messages

Remember that the digestive system, through its connection to the central nervous system (CNS), is primarily under the control of something called the enteric nervous system (ENS), which is capable of making autonomic decisions. Part of the visceral nervous system, the ENS also sends messages to the brain on topics related to digestion so that the brain can interpret and suggest appropriate behavior when necessary.

GI DIDN'T KNOW!

Contrary to popular belief, stress does not cause IBS. However, stressful thoughts and situations can definitely make it much worse.

For example, let's say that something you've eaten or medicine you have swallowed has caused you to feel the burning pain of acid reflux. An electrical message is sent to the brain requesting advice. The brain says "take an antacid" or "go see your doctor." You follow through on this behavior, and the problem goes away. Well, sort of. With a faulty electrical system, visceral messages continue to be sent even after the "pain" is over. "I'm still in pain," it communicates. On a similar note, the message being sent may be incorrectly amplified. For example, "I'm in pain" may end up being sent as "I'm really, really in a lot of pain here!" explaining why even minor stimuli can be gut wrenching. Interestingly, this visceral hypersensitivity is what may be responsible for the type of IBS that is pain predominant. But there's more.

A faulty electrical system can also wreak havoc with the normal digestive process. Miscommunication can cause the gut to contract too often, resulting in cramping and diarrhea, or it might cause the gut not to contract as it should, causing bloating and constipation. In fact, fluctuations of low-intensity and high-intensity signals can occur close together, which would explain why some IBS patients experience both diarrhea and a feeling of constipation within the same day.

Clearly, if this problem of faulty messages were the primary cause of IBS, it would have enormous implications for treatment—the brain-belly connection would have to be addressed more directly. It would explain why both antidepressants and *cognitive behavior therapy* (*CBT*) have been successful in obtaining positive results in some IBS sufferers. It may also explain why many people with IBS also suffer from conditions such as depression, fibromyalgia, chronic fatigue syndrome, and migraine headaches. In fact, very often people with a collection of chronic pain syndromes find that CBT is of tremendous help where other medications, including antidepressants, fail.

DEFINITION

Cognitive behavior therapy (CBT) is a short-term type of psychotherapy that helps the patient change thoughts and behaviors that result in or exacerbate emotional and physical symptoms. CBT may also include relaxation techniques.

Bacteria Gone Wild

Another suggested cause of IBS is a condition known as small intestinal bacteria overgrowth (SIBO). This condition occurs when intestinal flora, normally prevalent in the colon, set up shop in the small intestine and compete with you for nutrients. While doing so, they emit some nasty byproducts in this normally sterile environment, which can cause gas, bloating, vomiting, and diarrhea. Easily tested for with a hydrogen breath test (see Chapter 4) and usually treated with antibiotics, SIBO, although a probable cause for a small number of IBS cases, is not generally accepted as the primary cause due to a number of trials that have resulted in controversial data.

On the other hand, there appears to be a good amount of evidence that treating IBS with probiotics restores a healthy, natural balance to the digestive tract and helps to alleviate symptoms. We'll look at the role of probiotics for IBS patients, as well as other types of medication, when we talk about treatment options later in this chapter.

Other Causes?

Some researchers have suggested that IBS is actually a low-grade type of inflammatory bowel disease and is, consequently, autoimmune in nature, although there is little evidence to support this. However, one study indicated that IBS sufferers were 16 times more likely to develop IBD, which may be significant. Other studies have shown a link with conditions such as endometriosis and urinary bladder disease, but the nature of the connection is not known. It is also possible that IBS is caused by an as-yet-undiscovered active infection.

Foods as Triggers

Because food plays such a major role in digestive health, many people assume that what they eat has caused their condition. For diseases such as celiac disease, in which gluten is responsible for an inflammatory response and damage to the digestive tract, this is surely the case. However, there is no evidence that any specific foods cause IBS or that by avoiding them you will avoid developing the condition. On the other hand, some foods are known to trigger symptoms in people who already have IBS. These trigger foods include the following:

- Caffeine and alcohol
- Fatty and greasy foods

- Dairy products and fruit

- Artificial sweeteners such as sorbitol or xylitol

Getting a Diagnosis

When you begin your search for a diagnosis, you'll need a good amount of patience as well as an abundant supply of anecdotal information about your specific symptoms to help paint the clearest picture possible for your gastroenterologist. The greater the detail of your personal digestive history, the better equipped your doctor will be to conduct initial testing in the most fruitful and time-saving direction. It will also assist in eliminating other possible conditions that, as we've seen, are numerous and far reaching.

Tests of Exclusion

Because there are no specific laboratory or imaging tests that yield a diagnosis of IBS, your doctor will first need to exclude conditions that have IBS-like symptoms. Testing normally begins with blood work, including a complete blood count (CBC), a comprehensive metabolic panel (CMP), and a look at thyroid-stimulating hormone (TSH) levels. These tests help doctors rule out thyroid problems as the cause of your diarrhea or constipation and help to exclude gastrointestinal (GI) infections and ulcer disease, among other issues.

In particular, your doctor will also want to exclude the possibility of celiac disease by checking for specific antibodies to tissue transglutaminase (tTG) with an anti-tTG test—the common blood test for this condition. An upper endoscopy, perhaps with a biopsy, may be recommended as well to definitely discount celiac disease and any other conditions that may be reflected in tissue changes. Often a colonoscopy is also done to check for IBD or microscopic colitis (see Chapter 12) and to reassure the patient that the colon itself is not damaged. Finally, if small intestinal bacterial overgrowth is suspected, the doctor may order a breath or other test. In some cases, a stool sample may be checked for the presence of blood or mucus.

If your doctor believes that your initial testing has adequately eliminated the possibility of other conditions, he or she may recommend that you begin a treatment plan before being subjected to further costly or uncomfortable tests. However, if any red flags have come up either through initial testing or from your personal history, such as anemia, abdominal pain that does not go away after elimination, or nocturnal diarrhea, the doctor may order other diagnostic tests sooner rather than later. They may include a computed tomography (CT) scan or an MRI angiography to examine the abdominal blood flow.

More Imitators

As disheartening as it sounds, there are many, many more conditions and diseases that could be responsible for the symptoms of abdominal pain, diarrhea, and constipation. Testing for all of them is nearly impossible and not something you or your doctor should be eager to do. Rare diseases do occasionally occur in the average person and not just on medical TV shows, but unless you are exhibiting other specific chronic or unusual symptoms that might point to another explanation for your digestive problems, it's often best to begin a safe and sound treatment program to see if your symptoms improve. However, it may be worthwhile—especially if chronic pain is present—to seek the opinion of other specialists to determine if you may also be suffering from other chronic pain syndromes such as fibromyalgia, restless leg syndrome, chronic fatigue, or a condition referred to as *somatization disorder*, which would help dictate the course of your treatment.

DEFINITION

Somatization disorder, also called Briquet's syndrome, is a psychological condition in which physical symptoms mimic disease but no cause can be found.

Treating Irritable Bowel Syndrome

Once your doctor is satisfied that early testing has not turned up other explanations and is confident that IBS is the cause of your symptoms, he or she will recommend a treatment program. Although no treatment will cure IBS, the primary goal is to relieve as many of your symptoms as possible without adding any further discomfort as a result of the prescribed treatment. Recommendations are likely to target the predominant symptom or symptoms and to improve your overall digestive health.

If you haven't already begun to keep a food diary, this is something you should immediately do so that you and your doctor can note correlations between not only what you are eating, but when and under what circumstances. Although it may be a tedious prospect at first, with time it will become habit and may end up being the most important part of your IBS treatment plan.

When Diarrhea Dominates

Although occasional diarrhea responds well to over-the-counter remedies, continued use of these types of products is not a good idea. If taken for too long, they can result in chronic constipation, creating yet another uncomfortable symptom. As part of a treatment plan for IBS in which diarrhea predominates, your doctor will probably want to limit their use and instead will prescribe other types of medications and methods to control diarrhea, depending on its frequency and severity.

A common medication often prescribed for this variation of IBS is a type of antispasmodic drug to reduce spasms in the colon associated with cramping and diarrhea. Some antispasmodic medications are anticholinergics and work by blocking the neurotransmitter acetylcholine, which is released by the vagus nerve connecting the gut to the brain. In doing so, these medications act as a muscle relaxant and help to relieve both pain and cramping.

GULP!

Anticholinergics such as Levsin, Pamine, and Bentyl can cause a number of side effects, including dry mouth, drowsiness, and urination problems. In addition, you should not take these drugs if you suffer from glaucoma.

Peppermint oil, a natural antispasmodic, has shown to be extremely helpful as well and does not carry the side effects that other antispasmodic drugs often do. Unless acid reflux is a problem for you (peppermint can relax the lower esophageal sphincter, which encourages acid backup), peppermint oil capsules may be the safest choice.

In general, antispasmodics are taken 30 to 45 minutes before a meal to work optimally. For people with urgency-type diarrhea that comes on quickly following a meal or even before stressful situations, antispasmodic drugs can be particularly helpful in eliminating trepidation and restoring confidence and normalcy to an IBS sufferer's life.

Lotronex, a drug specifically designed for severe diarrhea-predominant IBS in women, was removed from the market in 2000 due to potential life-threatening side effects. In 2002, however, it was allowed to return with strict warnings, but its clinical use has not returned to previous levels.

When Constipation Is Chronic

Just as using over-the-counter antidiarrheal remedies is not a long-term solution, stimulant laxatives that help you cope with constipation are not recommended for extended use either. You and your doctor need to find a better way to relieve your chronic constipation, and one of the best and easiest ways to do so is to add more fiber to your diet (see Chapter 16). If you are not used to eating much fiber-rich food, introduce it into your diet slowly to prevent excess gas and bloating. Also, be sure to consume plenty of water, which will help reduce symptoms and encourage smooth bowel movements.

If you are unable to ingest an adequate amount of fiber through your diet, fiber supplements, often containing *psyllium*, may be part of your treatment plan. Adequate water intake is necessary with these as well. If excess bloating, gas, and cramping are still an issue, your doctor may recommend a newer type of laxative called Miralax, which works by keeping water in the bowel, resulting in softer stools. Previously only available by prescription, it is now available over the counter.

DEFINITION

Psyllium is a type of plant whose husks and seeds are used as a mild bulk laxative. Psyllium is often added to foods by manufacturers to increase fiber content and can also be bought as a supplement by consumers.

When your constipation is not adequately relieved with fiber or other nonprescription treatments, your doctor may suggest a prescribed medication called Amitiza (lubiprostone). Taken twice a day, it works by increasing fluid secretion in the small intestine to help with the passage of stool. It is not without side effects, however, which can include nausea, abdominal pain, and diarrhea, although if taken about 30 minutes after a meal, the nausea may be less severe.

Chronic constipation that does not respond to usual IBS treatment may require further investigation and medication. Sometimes the cause is due to slow motility, meaning that contractions of the digestive tract are, for some reason, greatly reduced. Often this happens as a result of other medications, particularly narcotics that notoriously cause severe constipation. Doctors often prescribe methylnaltrexone in this situation. Similarly, conditions such as scleroderma, advanced diabetes, or a rare metabolic disease called amyloidosis can cause reduced motility and may need to be addressed by a specialist.

GULP!

The drug tegaserod, marketed as Zelnorm, for constipation related to IBS was officially taken off the market in 2008 due to an increased risk of heart attack, stroke, and angina.

When Pain Prevails

Although both chronic diarrhea and constipation can certainly cause discomfort and pain, IBS that is primarily pain related is often treated somewhat differently. Many doctors prescribe some form of antidepressant to help with pain-predominant IBS. This treatment doesn't imply that you are clinically depressed, although IBS and its ongoing symptoms may definitely make you feel frustrated and depressed at times. The dosage of antidepressants often given to IBS sufferers is much lower than that prescribed specifically for depression and anxiety, but the treatment has been shown to reduce IBS pain by blocking signals to the brain. *Tricyclic antidepressants* such as Pamelor (often given for migraines) or Elavil are often prescribed. Other types of antidepressants, including Paxil or Cymbalta, have also been shown to provide IBS pain relief.

DEFINITION

Tricyclic antidepressants are the oldest class of antidepressant drugs. They work by blocking the re-uptake of neurotransmitters such as serotonin and norepinephrine.

Probably one of the most important ways you can help alleviate pain related to IBS, especially if you have other chronic pain issues, is to participate in cognitive behavior therapy (CBT). Many gastroenterologists are now recommending CBT for patients with IBS even if pain is not the predominant symptom because CBT has shown to be, along with other types of behavioral therapies including relaxation techniques, even more successful than medication for many people. If you go this route, locate a therapist who deals specifically with GI-related CBT and who will interact with your gastroenterologist as needed.

Although agreeing to this type of treatment may at first make you feel as if everyone thinks it really is "all in your mind," remember that the brain-gut connection is a very real, medically proven phenomenon and that much of what CBT accomplishes naturally is identical to what medicines may do for you artificially. Much study has indicated that these types of therapy can actually change brain chemistry and improve many health conditions.

More Help

All IBS sufferers may benefit from taking probiotics to restore healthy bacteria in the colon. Recent studies testing the effects of specific types of probiotics, including Lactobacillus plantarum and Bifidobacteria, have been particularly promising. In the past, the few people who even knew what a probiotic was had to seek high and low at health food stores. Now, however, supplements are readily available over the counter. Have your doctor recommend which product is best for you to try and how to work it into your treatment plan. There are many food sources of probiotics as well, which we'll be looking at in Part 5.

Relaxation techniques that relieve stress, such as yoga and meditation, can also help with IBS symptoms, and some alternative therapies have been shown to be beneficial as well (see Chapter 18). Even simple exercise, whether it be a nature walk or bicycle ride, helps bring oxygen into the colon to stimulate movement and improve brain chemistry to alleviate pain.

Finally, keeping current with your food diary is a good habit to continue even when your symptoms tend to subside. As you begin to feel better, you may want to add different types of foods to your diet to see how you react. For example, if you eliminated dairy products at first because of bloating and diarrhea but would like to try including them again, your handy diary will be able to record how you do and will help determine whether, indeed, you may be lactose intolerant. Often IBS sufferers are able to return to certain foods that caused distress before they received treatment.

The Least You Need to Know

- Irritable bowel syndrome (IBS) is a disorder that interferes with the normal functions of the colon but does not harm the intestines or cause colon cancer.
- The symptoms of IBS are abdominal pain and cramping, bloating, constipation, and diarrhea, often with one particular symptom predominating.
- The exact cause of IBS is unknown, but it may be due to an abnormal communication problem between the gut and brain.

- Stress and certain foods can trigger IBS symptoms.

- IBS is diagnosed by its symptoms and by the exclusion of other diseases through diagnostic testing.

- IBS can be controlled by a treatment plan that may include medication, dietary alterations, cognitive behavior therapy, and stress relief.

Polyps and Colon Cancer

In This Chapter

- All about colorectal polyps
- The connection between polyps and cancer
- When colon cancer is diagnosed

The health of our colons has been a hot topic in modern medicine. Not only are we aware of diseases and conditions that can affect the colon's function, such as Crohn's, colitis, and irritable bowel syndrome (IBS), but we are also more conscious than ever about the danger of developing colon cancer. Also called colorectal cancer, colon cancer is one of the top deadly cancers in America, but thanks to our awareness that may be changing. With more and more people getting routine colonoscopies, much of the cancer that may have previously gone undetected, and therefore untreated, is being discovered and eradicated.

Because almost 95 percent of colon cancer cases stem from polyps, a discussion of these types of growths is an important part of learning about colon cancer. This isn't to say that all polyps become cancerous. They do not. We'll also be looking in this chapter at the various types of polyps that may be encountered during a colonoscopy and how they differ from one another. We'll also explore the procedure known as polypectomy in which polyps are removed.

Once diagnosed, treating colon cancer depends on the stage at which it is detected and the range of its spread. We'll look at the current treatment plans normally recommended as well as the outlook for those who have been diagnosed. With early detection, colon cancer is no longer the death sentence it once was. Routine screening with a nod to family history, as well as a healthy diet and lifestyle, greatly help reduce the chances that your life or that of a family member is at risk from this common cancer.

What Are Polyps?

Colorectal *polyps* are small growths that form on the lining of the colon or rectum and that are most often benign but can sometimes become cancerous. Polyps in the colon are extremely common, and it is estimated that at least 50 percent of people over the age of 60 will have at least one.

> **DEFINITION**
>
> **Polyps** are fleshy, abnormal growths of tissue that may appear throughout the body on mucous membranes. The most common places to find polyps are the colon, rectum, stomach, small intestine, uterus, cervix, bladder, nose, and sinuses.

Types and Forms

Two main types of polyps are normally found in the colon:

- Hyperplastic

- Adenomatous

Hyperplastic polyps are benign, noncancerous growths resembling scar tissue, and they account for between 10 and 30 percent of all colorectal polyps that are found. About 70 percent of colon polyps found are adenomatous polyps—called adenomas—and these are also benign at the beginning. However, they have the ability to become malignant. Not all adenomatous polyps lead to cancer, but the majority of colon cancer cases have their start in adenomas.

> **GI DIDN'T KNOW!**
>
> Unlike the average polyp finding that may reveal three to five growths, people with rare genetic conditions such as familial adenomatous polyposis (FAP) may have hundreds or even thousands of polyps!

In addition, there are two other less common types of polyps that usually pose little danger of becoming cancerous. These two uncommon polyp types are …

- Inflammatory polyps that are associated with ulcerative colitis (UC) or Crohn's disease (CD), sometimes called pseudopolyps.

- Hamartomatous polyps, which result from mutations. These could, when associated with rare, often inherited diseases, sometimes become cancerous.

Polyps are also described by their shape. Sessile polyps look like spilled paint and are normally only slightly raised from the surface of the colon lining. Pedunculated polyps look like little mushrooms and are attached to the colon lining by a narrow stalk.

Does Size Matter?

Although colon polyps can certainly appear as large as a golf ball or even bigger, most are smaller than the size of a pea, especially when found during a routine colonoscopy. The risk that a polyp contains signs of cancer appears to be directly related to its size. This is particularly important when evaluating adenomas.

The general rule of thumb is that polyps measuring 1 centimeter or larger begin to carry a certain percentage of risk. The larger the polyp, the greater the chance that precancerous or malignant cells may be present. Specifically, here's the breakdown:

- Less than 1 cm = 2 percent risk

- 1 to 2 cm = 10 to 20 percent risk

- Greater than 2 cm = 30 to 50 percent risk

GULP!

Possibly the largest colon polyp discovered to date was recently found in a middle-aged man in Korea. It measured 9.5 cm across—about the size of a large navel orange—and was benign.

Who's the Villain?

For the most part, adenomatous polyps are the ones to look out for when screening for colon cancer, although your gastroenterologist will not be able to determine whether a polyp seen during the colonoscopy is adenomatous or hyperplastic until it is removed and examined by a pathologist under a microscope. Once a polyp is determined to be an adenoma, it will be further classified into one of three types according to its appearance: tubular, tubulovillous, or villous. These subtypes also carry their own risk of malignancy:

- Tubular adenomas: 5 percent risk

- Tubulovillous adenomas: 20 percent risk

- Villous adenomas: 40 percent risk

Tubular adenomas are by far the most common, and villous adenomas are considered the most aggressive. Recently, another type known as a sessile serrated adenoma has also been implicated as being potentially precancerous, perhaps carrying the most malignant risk of all polyps. Usually quite flat and difficult to see (as well as remove), gastroenterologists have made a particular point of looking for these as well during a polyp screening.

Polyp Causes and Risks

Polyps are the result of abnormal cell growth, which can be caused by a variety of interacting factors. The main factors are genetic and environmental. Some people are simply more apt to develop polyps and, potentially, colon cancer because of their genetic approach to cell division. Others may be prone to developing polyps because of their diet and lifestyle choices. Unfortunately, as we age, years of wear and tear on the colon can also be a factor that in many cases is unavoidable, so sheer luck can also play a role in the development of polyps.

Family Factors

Under normal circumstances, healthy cells grow and divide in an orderly fashion throughout the body. In the colon, this is controlled by two broad groups of genes. If an inherited mutation is present in any of these genes, cells may continue to divide even when not needed and begin to create polyps. If mutation continues as the cell division continues, the tissue starts acting separately from the body's natural road-blocks to tumors, leaving the door open for cancer formation. In rare and extreme cases, some people may develop polyps and colon cancer at a relatively early age, sometimes accompanied by other cancers—of the uterus, stomach, or pancreas. The most common inherited form of colon cancer, accounting for up to 7 percent of all cases, is heredity nonpolyposis colorectal cancer (HNPCC), once known as Lynch syndrome. This type carries such a great risk that patients with proven inheritance may elect to have their colons removed rather than opt for annual colonoscopies. However, most inherited tendencies toward polyp formation are not as dramatic.

Having a sibling, parent, or child with colon polyps or colon cancer can certainly raise your risk. If more than one close relative has also experienced polyps and cancer, your risk is even greater. Not all family cases are necessarily inherited, however, because a shared environment with exposure to *carcinogens* or the same poor diet could also cause multiple family members to be susceptible.

DEFINITION

Carcinogens are substances or agents that increase the risk of cancer. Common carcinogens include radiation, asbestos, and tobacco smoke.

Your family's ethnic background and race also play a role. African Americans and Ashkenazi Jews of Eastern European descent are more likely to develop polyps and colon cancer than others. It is sometimes recommended that screening begin at age 45 rather than the usual 50 for people in these groups, as well as African Americans. It's also often prudent to screen early if a close family member has had colon cancer at an early age—about 10 years before your relative's onset.

You Are What You Eat

More to the point, you are what you eat, drink, and smoke. There is sufficient evidence to suggest that a diet high in red meat (particularly if high in saturated fat), charred meats, and processed meats can increase your polyp and cancer risk. Heavy beer consumption has also been linked to an increase of polyp formation. If you smoke while you're swigging your beer, your chances increase even more. In fact, smokers are 20 percent more likely to develop colon cancer than nonsmokers. Although beer is often cited as the main culprit, all forms of alcoholic beverages, if consumed in excess, can add to your chances of developing polyps. There appears also to be a connection between diabetes, obesity, lack of exercise, and the consumption of a high-fat diet.

It was once believed that a diet high in fiber prevented polyp formation, but recent studies have somewhat discredited previous ones. This isn't to say that a healthy diet that includes fiber found in fruits, vegetables, and whole grains should be discounted because there is good evidence that our general health receives a boost from eating these types of foods. The healthier we are, the less likely we will be to contract many types of diseases, including colon cancer. Although fiber may not be preventive in a direct sense, it is still an excellent part of maintaining digestive health (see Chapter 16).

What *does* seem to prevent polyp formation is supplementing your diet with calcium and vitamin D. According to a study published in the *Journal of the National Cancer Institute*, people taking calcium supplements of 1,200 milligrams per day were less likely to be diagnosed with colorectal cancer. Exactly how calcium does this is not known, but it may play a part in inhibiting the growth of polyps. Taking a low-dose aspirin once a day may also help to keep polyps at bay, but be sure to speak with your physician before adding any supplements (including aspirin) to your diet, as they can sometimes create their own set of problems in certain people.

Checking for Polyps

If you have colorectal polyps, it is unlikely that you are displaying any symptoms. On rare occasions, especially if they are large, polyps can cause you to have some digestive problems that are similar to many other GI conditions. Any of these digestive issues would certainly warrant investigation:

- Rectal bleeding
- Blood in the stool
- Narrowing of the stool
- Diarrhea or constipation
- Cramping and abdominal pain

Because of the usual lack of symptoms, screening for polyps is highly recommended once you reach the age of 50. If you have a higher risk of developing colon cancer because of family history or a chronic disease such as ulcerative colitis or Crohn's, testing even earlier is recommended, if not a must.

Colonoscopy Is Critical

Not long ago, probing for polyps simply involved checking for blood in the stool and having a sigmoidoscopy (see Chapter 4). These less-than-satisfactory methods of testing failed to detect many polyps and potential cases of colon cancer. Today, the colonoscopy is the gold standard for screening and is the best chance you have of discovering polyp growth and preventing colon cancer.

We discussed what to expect during your colonoscopy in Chapter 4, but it's worth emphasizing the importance of your preparation for the test. Unless your colon is pristine and free of all fecal matter, your doctor may not be able to discover all polyps, if they exist. A good cleanout also affects how well you feel after the procedure and how quickly you are up and about once again. Preparation procedures are continually being improved and updated, so even if you think you know the drill from previous colonoscopies, study the current material your doctor's office provides to ensure you are doing everything correctly.

Removing Polyps

Most polyps found during a colonoscopy are immediately removed with a procedure called a polypectomy. Small polyps (less than 5 mm) are generally removed with biopsy forceps, a tool that looks a bit like an alligator clip. Sometimes an electric current is passed through the forceps. This is called a "hot biopsy," and it increases the chances of getting the whole polyp from the base and also reduces the possibility of bleeding. A "cold biopsy," without an electric current, might be done on particularly small polyps (less than 3 mm), reducing the chance of perforation of the colon, a rare outcome in either case.

Slightly larger polyps are probably removed using a snare—a metal lasso-type instrument—also with an electrical current. To assist removal, sometimes a sterile saline solution tinged with blue is injected so that the doctor can see the outline of the polyp—particularly helpful when dealing with flat or only slightly raised ones. For larger polyps, it may take several sessions to be sure the entire growth has been removed. In these instances, a procedure known as argon plasma coagulation (APC) might also be performed. This involves burning any residual pieces of the polyps that have been removed.

GULP!

Poorly cleaned-out colons with residual fecal matter could prove to have dynamic consequences. Bacterial fermentation coupled with argon gas used in an APC procedure has, in rare instances, caused the colon to literally explode.

Following Up

If your colonoscopy results in a "clean exam" with no sign of polyps, you'll probably be advised to return for another screening in 10 years, although some physicians are now recommending intervals of 5 years, just to be on the safe side. The 10-year rule stems from the belief that most colon cancers take 10 years to develop from normal cells to polyp to cancer. But recent studies have revealed that some people have been diagnosed with colon cancer just five years after a clean colonoscopy.

If polyps are found during your colonoscopy, you'll be advised to return for a follow-up exam, depending on the type and number of polyps you had. Because the discovery of polyps increases your chance of having them again, your doctor will want to keep an eye on your colon and may suggest a repeat colonoscopy within a couple of years. If the polyps were of the villous type or if there were more than five with any being over 1 centimeter in size, a follow-up will be required in a year. If a polyp requires more than one session to be removed or requires multiple attempts during a single session, follow-up will be recommended within three to six months.

Diagnosing Colon Cancer

If colon cancer is to be a part of your life, early detection through routine screening is by far the best way to discover and eradicate it. Unfortunately, not every colon cancer patient has been vigilant about colonoscopy screening, or someone may have a particularly aggressive form of cancer that is diagnosed when certain symptoms have already begun to appear. These symptoms, also common to other digestive disorders, may include the following:

- A change in bowel habits, including consistency and frequency, as well as pencil-thin stool

- Rectal bleeding or blood in the stool

- Persistent abdominal pain, cramps, or gas

- Weakness or fatigue

- Weight loss

If you present with these types of symptoms with no history of screening or without a recent screening, no doubt a thorough physical examination, blood work, and, of course, a colonoscopy will be advised to determine the cause. If polyps are found and cancer is suspected, a biopsy will be done as well as further evaluation of the state of the cancer, with treatment beginning right away.

Location and Spread

Colon cancer can affect any part of the colon, from the cecum at the beginning to the rectum at the end. Sometimes when the cancer is limited to the rectum, it is referred to specifically as rectal cancer and often requires slightly different treatment approaches. Otherwise, colon cancer is generally diagnosed and staged according to the degree to which it has spread. To determine the extent of the spread, a computed tomography (CT) scan and/or endoscopic ultrasound (EUS) is conducted. A blood test that checks for the elevation of specific proteins related to the spread of the cancer is also done.

The actual staging of the cancer cannot be determined without surgery. Treatment does not begin until staging is complete. However, patients with rectal cancer often receive radiation therapy prior to surgery to help relieve symptoms and shrink the tumor.

If the cancer is small and localized in a polyp, your doctor may be able to remove it completely during a colonoscopy. If the pathologist determines that the cancer in the polyp doesn't involve the base—where the polyp is attached to the intestinal wall— then there's a good chance that the cancer has been completely eliminated. Still, some doctors may wish to remove the section of the colon where the polyp was found to be completely safe, in which case surgery is necessary.

For most other cases with greater polyp or cancer involvement, if imaging and other testing indicate there has been no spread beyond the colon, surgery will likely be planned, and samples of tissue and nearby lymph nodes will be taken to help determine the appropriate therapy and the actual staging of the cancer. If cancer is found on a biopsy, then a CT scan helps stage the tumor. If it appears that cancer is in the liver, you may not get surgery right away as options are explored. If cancer is found in lymph nodes, then you'll likely get chemotherapy.

Staging Colon Cancer

Like other forms of cancer, staging is done to determine the best treatment as well as to give an educated prognosis. There are a number of different staging systems that are often specific to the cancer involved. In the past, systems known as the Dukes and the Astler-Coller were used for colon cancer, but they are less precise than the tumor/node/metastasis (TNM) system, which is the standard one used today.

The TNM system describes three key pieces of information:

- "T" indicates how far the primary tumor has grown into the wall of the intestine and/or into nearby areas

- "N" describes the extent of spread to nearby lymph nodes

- "M" indicates whether the cancer has spread, or metastasized, to other organs of the body

Numbers are then assigned following each letter to provide more details about each of these factors. The numbers 0 through 4 indicate increasing severity, and sometimes the letter "X" is added if an assessment cannot be made because certain information is unavailable.

For example, you might receive a TNM staging that looks like this: "T1, N0, M0," meaning that the cancer has grown through the inner lining (T1), but has not spread to lymph nodes (N0) or distant sites (M0).

Once these numbers are determined, an actual stage grouping can be assigned to your case which will assist in making treatment decisions. Stage grouping designations are Roman numerals (plus 0).

- Stage 0: The cancer is in the earliest stage, meaning it has not grown beyond the inner layer (mucosa) of the colon or rectum. This stage of cancer may also be called "carcinoma in situ."

- Stage I: The cancer has grown through the mucosa but has not spread beyond the colon wall or rectum.

- Stage II: The cancer has grown into or through the wall of the colon or rectum but has not spread to nearby lymph nodes.

- Stage III: The cancer has invaded nearby lymph nodes but is not yet affecting other parts of the body.

- Stage IV: The cancer has spread to distant sites—other organs such as the liver or lungs.

- Recurrent: The cancer has come back after treatment in the colon, rectum, or other part of the body.

So in the preceding TNM example, the stage grouping for "T1, N0, M0" would be stage I.

TUMMY TIP

In some instances, your cancer may fall between two categories, and the diagnosis may be very much a judgment call by your doctor. Although many patients don't ask to see their pathology reports or have the staging process explained to them, you should consider doing so because it is important in understanding your situation, especially if you decide to seek a second opinion.

Cancer Treatment and Prognosis

Treatment options for colon cancer are similar to those of other cancers and include surgery, chemotherapy, radiation, and sometimes targeted drug therapy. Depending on the stage of the cancer, your doctor may recommend two or more of these treatments either together or one after another. In addition to the stage, other factors taken into consideration include your overall health, the likely side effects of the treatment, and the probability of curing the disease, extending life, or relieving symptoms.

Surgical Procedures

Surgery for colon cancer is performed either laparoscopically or by local incision of the abdomen. Laparoscopic procedures are far less invasive and are possible with some types of early stage colon cancers. It is the same procedure typically used to remove the gallbladder (see Chapter 13) and can be just as curative as traditional surgery. Instead of making one long incision in the abdomen, the surgeon makes several smaller incisions. Special long instruments are inserted through these incisions to remove part of the colon and lymph nodes. One of these instruments has a small video camera on the end, which allows the surgeon to see inside the intestine. Once the diseased part of the colon has been freed, one of the incisions is made larger to allow for its removal.

If the cancer is invasive but treatable (or simply beyond the possibilities of a laparoscopic procedure), traditional, open-abdominal surgery will take place to remove the affected part of the colon. This is referred to as a colectomy or a segmental resection because the surgeon is often able to reconnect the healthy portions of your colon or rectum. Depending on the location of the cancer, sometimes a partial or full proctocolectomy—removal of both colon and rectum—is necessary. If that occurs, the surgeon then performs an ileostomy to create an opening in the wall of your abdomen from a portion of the remaining bowel for the elimination of body waste into a special bag. Referred to as a colostomy, sometimes it is only temporary, but in certain cases it may be permanent.

If the cancer is quite advanced and has spread to other organs, usually surgery will not be recommended except for *palliative* purposes. The exception to this is when only the liver has shown signs of metastasis that are limited in nature, in which case removing these lesions, as well as any colon tumors that may exist, can often improve a patient's prognosis.

DEFINITION

Palliative care is any kind of treatment that reduces disease symptoms but is not expected to be curative. The goal is to prevent and relieve suffering and, in the case of colon cancer, might involve surgery to remove a blockage or stop chronic bleeding.

Radiation and Chemotherapy

Radiation therapy uses high-energy rays or particles to destroy cancer cells and may be part of the treatment recommended for either colon or rectal cancer. Because chemotherapy can make radiation therapy more effective in many instances, these two treatments are often used together.

For rectal cancer in particular, radiation therapy is usually given along with chemotherapy to help prevent the cancer from coming back where the tumor started. Giving radiation before surgery, however, is often done as well to avoid complications such as scar formation that can interfere with bowel movements or to reduce the size of tumors in the rectum to make surgery easier. When therapy is given before surgery, it is called neoadjuvant treatment, as opposed to therapy given after surgery, which is known as adjuvant treatment.

Chemotherapy may also be used at different times (neoadjuvant or adjuvant) to treat colon and rectal cancers, but it is most often given following surgery. Adjuvant chemotherapy can increase the survival rate for patients with some stages of colon cancer and rectal cancer. Because a small number of cancer cells may not have been removed by surgery or may have escaped from the primary tumor and settled in other parts of the body, postsurgical chemotherapy is often a standard part of treatment. The hope is that the chemotherapy will kill these cells wherever they may be. Treatment may be provided intravenously or in pill form, and often a combination of two different drugs is used.

As researchers have learned more about the gene and protein changes in cells that cause cancer, they have been able to develop drugs that specifically target these changes. These targeted drugs work differently than standard chemotherapy drugs and often have different, sometimes less severe, side effects. They are most often used either along with chemotherapy or by themselves if chemotherapy is no longer working. They are typically reserved for patients with advanced colon cancer. Some people benefit from targeted drug therapies; others do not. Research continues to examine the best way to administer this type of therapy and under what circumstances its use is most appropriate.

Surviving Colon Cancer

Because many cases of colon cancer are now detected during routine screenings, the survival rate has significantly improved in recent years. In the United States, the overall five-year survival rate after initial diagnosis is estimated at 62 percent. When caught in its early stage, however, colon cancer patients have a survival rate as high as 93 percent. These statistics demonstrate the extreme importance of colonoscopy screening.

GI DIDN'T KNOW!

The decline in colon cancer cases is contributing to a general decline in cancer rates in the United States, according to a recent study. Credit goes to the colonoscopy, the only medical screening test that not only detects but actually reduces the number of cancer cases through polyp removal, making it an invaluable therapeutic as well as diagnostic tool.

There appears to be a positive connection between survival rates and exercise for all stages of colon cancer. One study revealed that moderate exercise increased early survival rates by as much as 55 percent in patients with stage III cancer, while another study, which included patients with stages I, II, and III, revealed a 50 percent increase. When it comes to *preventing* colon cancer, exercise can decrease your risk by at least 40 percent.

The Least You Need to Know

- A colorectal polyp is a growth on the inner lining of the colon or rectum and can appear raised or flat.
- Most polyps are benign and are removed during routine colonoscopy screenings by a procedure called a polypectomy.
- Some polyps, particularly of the adenomatous type, can become cancerous.
- Some people are more likely than others to develop polyps and colon cancer due to genetic factors as well as diet and lifestyle.
- The best way to avoid colon cancer is by having routine colonoscopies beginning at the age of 50, or younger if you are at higher risk.
- Colon cancer, especially when found in its earliest stages, can be successfully treated through a combination of surgery and therapy, including chemotherapy and radiation.

Other Lower GI Conditions

Chapter 12

In This Chapter

- Diverticulitis and other colon conditions
- More inflammatory bowel disorders
- Miscellaneous GI-related problems

We've covered all the main conditions and diseases that are related to your lower gastrointestinal (GI) digestive health in the previous chapters, but there are a few more that are worth a quick rundown. Although it's impossible to mention everything, this chapter will provide a brief understanding of some of the conditions that might affect you.

Diverticulosis and diverticulitis often cause a lot of confusion, so we'll spell out what you need to know about these relatively common conditions that affect us as we age. We'll also take a look at some lesser-known, colon-related diseases that can cause uncomfortable symptoms and require medical attention. These include ischemic colitis and a few types of inflammatory bowel conditions that we haven't touched on before.

Finally, we'll take a look at the problem of hemorrhoids, which can be the cause of much annoyance and irritation. We'll consider somewhat-related occurrences called anal fissures that can interfere with normal bowel habits by causing pain as well as bleeding. We'll finish with a quick discussion of appendicitis because the appendix—technically anyway—is considered part of the digestive system. Although the contribution of the appendix to the digestive team is pretty much nil, when the appendix flares up, you need to take note of it, so symptoms and treatment are included here as well.

Diverticulosis and Diverticulitis

These relatively common conditions that affect the colon (and sometimes the small bowel) often cause more confusion at first than the actual symptoms. A brief lesson in medical Latin will help. Here's the gist:

- A diverticulum is an outpouching of the colon lining, usually about the size of a marble.

- When you have more than one diverticulum (pouch), they are called diverticula (pouches).

- The condition of having diverticula is called diverticulosis.

- When diverticula become inflamed, the condition is called diverticulitis.

- Diverticulosis and diverticulitis together are referred to as diverticular disease.

If you haven't already noticed, the common root word is *divert*, meaning to turn aside or deflect from a path or course. Imagine a detour, which is what these outpouchings often look like during imaging tests. Diverticula are also sometimes referred to as herniations within the colon, but are not, in essence, true hernias. Most diverticula appear in the sigmoid colon, the last segment of the large intestine. Because most diverticula are believed to be caused by excess straining of the bowel to defecate, often as a result of constipation, this location makes sense. This is the area of the colon where there is the least amount of liquid left after digested matter has made its way through the intestinal tract and been thoroughly processed.

Excess pressure can cause naturally weak spots in the colon to bulge out and form diverticula. Although diverticulosis rarely causes symptoms, occasional mild abdominal pain may be felt in the lower-left quadrant, as well as bloating and constipation. Because symptoms are usually rare, most diverticula are incidentally found during routine colonoscopy screenings or tests for other diseases.

Probable Causes

The primary cause of diverticula development is simple aging. It's estimated that half of all Americans age 60 to 80 have them and that just about everyone over the age of 80 will have at least one. You can develop diverticula at a younger age, but this is unusual unless there are other health complications that encourage their formation, such as certain kidney diseases or conditions that weaken the body's connective tissue, such as *Marfan syndrome.*

> **DEFINITION**
>
> **Marfan syndrome** is an inherited disorder that allows connective tissue in the body to stretch abnormally, often resulting in an extremely long face and limbs, among other traits. Until recently it was believed that Abraham Lincoln suffered from Marfan syndrome, but it is more likely that an endocrine disorder called Sipple's syndrome caused his characteristic features.

Another cause of diverticulosis is diet. Interestingly, diverticular disease is rare in places such as Africa and Asia, where people routinely eat a high-fiber diet. Here in America, as well as most of Europe, low fiber is unfortunately the norm, and this lack may play a critical role in the actual formation of diverticula. In fact, diverticular disease was first noted in the United States in the early 1900s, when processed foods—notoriously low in fiber—were introduced into the American diet.

When we eat lots of fiber, it not only bulks up the stool but allows it to absorb moisture, making bowel movements softer and easier to pass. Low-fiber food has the opposite effect, resulting in smaller and more compact stool. Muscles of the colon must apply more pressure in order to move it along. A lack of fiber combined with resulting constipation and straining to pass stool is probably responsible for the majority of diverticula that develop. Add our sedentary lifestyle and propensity toward obesity, and you have a country full of perfect candidates for diverticulosis.

Inflammatory Symptoms

As many as 25 percent of people with diverticulosis develop diverticulitis. Diverticulitis occurs when diverticula become inflamed or infected and is also when pain becomes a primary symptom. Sometimes sudden and severe, abdominal pain can also be experienced as mild at first but worsening over time. In addition, the following other symptoms may begin to appear:

- A change in bowel habits, particularly after a straining episode
- Diarrhea
- Constipation

- Fever

- Nausea and vomiting

- Rectal bleeding

Exactly what causes diverticula to become inflamed and infected is not entirely known. In the past, doctors thought that nuts, seeds, popcorn, and corn played a role in causing diverticulitis by getting trapped in diverticula. However, recent research has found that these foods are not to blame. Instead, it could be that the thin lining of the outpouching may simply burst because of excessive straining during defecation, allowing bacteria to leak out and cause infection. It may also be that a narrowing of the opening reduces blood supply to the area and causes inflammation or allows bacteria and fecal matter to become trapped.

GULP!

Although diverticulitis is usually considered a disease affecting older adults, doctors report an increase in cases in younger adults, particularly those with abdominal obesity.

Diverticular Complications

Diverticulitis can lead to a number of complications, including abscesses, fistulas (see Chapter 9), perforations, leakage, and blockages. Abscesses may require draining to avoid ruptures that could release pus and cause damage to colon tissue or even *peritonitis*. Fistulas can spread infection to other organs, particularly the bladder and urinary tract. Even small perforations can leak contents of the colon into the abdominal cavity, while scarring caused by infected diverticula may cause partial or even total blockage.

DEFINITION

Peritonitis is inflammation of the lining of the abdominal cavity (peritoneum) and can occur when inflamed or infected diverticula rupture and spill intestinal contents into the abdominal cavity. It requires immediate medical attention and can be fatal if not treated.

Diverticular bleeding can be a serious complication as well, with large amounts of blood loss and the need for possible surgery. A burst blood vessel in a diverticulum usually causes the bleeding and may be the result of vessel clogging and fragility caused by certain bacteria, or the use of certain medications such as nonsteroidal anti-inflammatory drugs (NSAIDs). Sometimes bleeding will stop by itself and not require treatment, but in all cases seek immediate medical attention.

Diagnosing Diverticulitis

Diverticulitis is usually diagnosed during an acute attack. Because the location of the pain and many of the other symptoms are similar to a number of conditions, your doctor will want to rule out other possible causes, including the following:

- Pelvic inflammatory disease

- Inflammatory bowel disease (IBD)

- Ischemic colitis

- Ovarian or colon cancer

- Irritable bowel syndrome (IBS)

If pain more generally appears in the lower abdominal region or even the right side, the doctor may want to consider appendicitis as well.

Tests for diverticulitis usually include a thorough physical exam, checking for tenderness in the abdominal area, blood work to show signs of infection, and a computed tomography (CT) scan to visualize any inflamed or infected pouches in the colon. Usually a colonoscopy is not done until six to eight weeks after treatment, as it may increase the risk of complications. Depending on your diagnosis as well as your ongoing symptoms, treatment may be decided and administered during a hospital stay or at home.

Treatment and Prevention

Mild cases of diverticulitis, even when an abscess may be present, can often be treated on an outpatient basis with antibiotics and instructions for bed rest and a temporary liquid or low-fiber diet. More severe cases often require a several-day hospital stay for intravenously administered antibiotics and for time for the colon to rest.

Acute or recurrent attacks of diverticulitis sometimes require surgery. Normally when surgery is recommended, the affected part of the colon is removed and the remaining sections joined—called a bowel resection—not unlike the surgery sometimes performed for Crohn's disease (CD) or colon cancer. In advanced cases a colectomy, removal of the entire colon, may be necessary, particularly if there is danger of recurrent bleeding or an emergency exists.

After an attack of diverticulitis subsides and after you have had a period of time eating a low-fiber or liquid diet in order to allow the colon to rest, reintroducing fiber into your daily eating routine will be of utmost importance. Your ultimate goal will be to eat a diet high in fiber (see Chapter 17) and to drink plenty of water as well. Doing so will help prevent further attacks and complications while keeping more diverticula from forming. It will be equally important to avoid straining during visits to the bathroom. Once you are eating lots of fiber-rich foods, straining will probably no longer be necessary.

Ischemic Colitis

Ischemic colitis is a disorder in which the colon becomes inflamed or damaged because of reduced or impaired blood flow. This reduced flow can occur abruptly, or it may develop gradually over time. Because of the low flow of blood, the colon may begin to starve and die. The areas of the colon that are normally involved with ischemic colitis are what physicians refer to as the "watershed" locations, which generally have the least blood supply anyway: the rectosigmoid junction, a region in the lower colon where the twisting part of the colon (sigmoid) joins the rectum, and the splenic flexure at the end of the transverse colon near the spleen.

You may be more familiar with the term *ischemia* in relation to heart disease, and in fact, people with coronary artery disease are often at greater risk of developing the chronic type of this colitis. But ischemic colitis can also be a result of something specific interrupting the blood supply to the colon, such as a blood clot, often the cause of acute attacks. It is also possible that infections involving bacteria such as *E. coli*, as well as a virus or parasite, could trigger ischemic colitis.

DEFINITION

Ischemia is the insufficient supply of blood to an organ or body part, typically the heart but also seen in the brain, intestines, kidneys, legs, and feet. Often the buildup of plaque in the arteries (atherosclerosis) is the cause.

Related Risks

In some instances, ischemic colitis is related to other medical conditions or circumstances. They might include the following:

- Vasculitis—inflammation of the blood vessels
- Diabetes mellitus (type 2)
- Hernias
- Low blood pressure
- Easy blood clotting
- Colon cancer
- Prior abdominal surgery
- Radiation treatment to the abdomen

In addition, the overuse of some medications has been associated with ischemic colitis, including laxatives like Dulcolax and some decongestants. Birth control pills and estrogen replacement therapy have also been shown to create a slight risk.

Age plays a large role as well, with most cases diagnosed in older adults. In fact, 90 percent of cases occur in people over the age of 60. When younger adults are affected, there is usually a good chance that vasculitis or a blood-clotting abnormality is the cause.

Signs and Symptoms

The following are the most common signs and symptoms of ischemic colitis:

- Abdominal pain, tenderness, or cramping, usually in the lower-left side, coming on suddenly or gradually
- Low-grade fever
- Bright red or maroon-colored blood in the stool or even passage of blood without stool, following abdominal pain
- A feeling of urgency to defecate
- Diarrhea

- Nausea

- Vomiting

GULP!

When signs and symptoms of ischemic colitis affect the right side of the colon, including the cecum and ascending colon, a potentially life-threatening condition called mesenteric ischemia, affecting the small bowel, may be the cause. This cut-off of blood flow can quickly cause small intestinal tissue death and usually requires immediate surgery.

Diagnostic Testing and Treatment

A colonoscopy (see Chapter 4) is the definitive test for ischemic colitis. The test allows your doctor to look for evidence of inflammation as well as to rule out other causes of your symptoms such as diverticulitis and IBD. Because swelling and bleeding can often occur under the colon lining with ischemic colitis, a biopsy is usually done as well so that colon tissue can be examined in the laboratory for this typical sign.

In addition, blood work checks for signs of elevated white blood cells, which are often seen with this condition. Your doctor may also refer you to a *hematologist* to check for blood-clotting issues. A stool sample may be taken to exclude an infection caused by bacteria or microorganisms that can sometimes be confused with ischemic colitis. An abdominal MRI may also be performed to view blood vessels and look for blockages.

DEFINITION

A **hematologist** is a physician who specializes in the study of blood and blood-related disorders.

Surprisingly, many cases of ischemic colitis require little treatment, as the condition often resolves on its own within a few days without need for hospitalization. Medications to keep your blood pressure normal may be prescribed to facilitate blood flow to the colon. Antibiotics may be prescribed as well. Once the inflammation has subsided, a follow-up colonoscopy may be recommended to check your progress in six to eight weeks.

In more severe cases, a hospital stay may be necessary if prolonged diarrhea has caused dehydration and/or you are unable to eat on your own. Surgery may be recommended in some cases to remove the affected part of the colon. When ischemic colitis becomes chronic and there are complications such as gangrene, perforations, strictures, or persistent bleeding, surgery likely will be required.

Other Inflammatory Bowel Conditions

Although Crohn's and ulcerative colitis (UC) are the main forms of IBD (see Chapter 9), there are other types of inflammatory conditions that are far less common but worth a quick review. Just about all types of IBD and infectious colitis cause the classic symptoms of an inflamed digestive tract with watery diarrhea and abdominal pain. Each type, however, has a different cause, often affecting a different group of people and carrying with it a variety of potential complications as well as treatment approaches.

Microscopic Colitis

This form of IBD typically affects middle-age females and is associated with a higher incidence of autoimmune disorders such as rheumatoid arthritis, diabetes, and celiac disease. It has also been associated with the use of NSAIDs, proton pump inhibitors (PPIs) used to treat GERD (see Chapter 5), and selective serotonin reuptake inhibitors such as Zoloft, used in the treatment of depression.

> **GI DIDN'T KNOW!**
>
> Behçet's syndrome is a rare type of IBD that creates exaggerated inflammation in blood vessels throughout the body, often affecting the eye, mouth, and genital area as well as the digestive tract. Because it is more common in the Middle East and Asia, it is sometimes referred to as Silk Road Disease.

In addition to chronic watery diarrhea, the other primary feature of microscopic colitis is a normal colonoscopy, but with biopsy results that indicate inflammatory cells only visible under a microscope—thus the name. There are two subcategories of microscopic colitis: collagenous colitis and lymphocytic colitis. These are differentiated by whether or not a thickened *collagen* layer is present in the lining of the colon.

> **DEFINITION**
>
> **Collagen** is the main protein found in connective tissue, providing it with strength and flexibility. Although usually discussed in relation to skin and aging, collagen is present throughout the body.

Treatment is usually a course of budesonide to reduce inflammation, the same steroid used to treat CD. This medication acts primarily in the digestive tract and is less likely to cause numerous side effects. Symptoms can be managed with over-the-counter medications such as Imodium or Pepto-Bismol. The majority of patients recover from their diarrhea, and any inflammatory abnormalities present are almost always resolved, making microscopic colitis a much less severe condition than other forms of IBD.

Clostridium Difficile Colitis

A type of infectious colitis, *Clostridium difficile* colitis is a growing concern in the medical community. Caused by the *Clostridium difficile* bacterium, this disease can easily and quickly spread in hospitals and other health facilities. Unfortunately, studies have indicated that a more virulent strain may be developing.

Once believed to be the exclusive result of antibiotics (such as clindamycin and levaquin) killing off healthy bacteria and in turn encouraging these nasty bacteria to flourish, more and more cases are now being seen that are unrelated. In particular, the elderly and people with compromised immune systems appear to be highly susceptible to *Clostridium difficile* colitis, as well as those who have had recent surgery. Cases vary in severity from mild diarrhea to extreme bloody diarrhea that could even result in toxic megacolon (see Chapter 9). A diagnosis is easily made using a stool sample to check for the presence of *Clostridium difficile* toxins. Sometimes healthy individuals show evidence of the toxin as well, suggesting that some people are protected from certain strains. Treatment usually involves specific types of antibiotics targeted at the digestive tract, such as metronidazole or vancomycin, an antibiotic once referred to as a drug of last resort.

GULP!

Another last resort once used to treat *Clostridium difficile* infections is fecal bacteriotherapy, in which feces are acquired from a healthy family member and made into an enema in an attempt to restore the patient's bacterial balance in the colon. Although some sources show a 95 percent success rate, this therapy is rarely used today.

Hemorrhoids and Fissures

Often the source of many a joke, hemorrhoids are no laughing matter. Sometimes referred to as "piles," hemorrhoids are swollen and inflamed veins in the rectum and anus. It is estimated that by the age of 50, about half of the population has experienced the itching, discomfort, and bleeding that often signals their presence.

Hemorrhoids are usually associated with constipation and straining during bowel movements, both of which increase pressure on the hemorrhoid veins. This pressure is also why pregnant women often develop them, as do obese individuals and those who sit for long periods of time.

A Pile of Symptoms

Symptoms of hemorrhoids depend on whether they are internal or external. Because internal ones are located in the area of the rectum that lacks pain receptors, most people do not know they even have them until they see the tell-tale sign of bright red blood on stool, toilet paper, or in the toilet bowl. Although this symptom is often alarming, rarely does hemorrhoid bleeding indicate a serious complication.

 GULP!

Don't always assume that painless bleeding from the rectum is automatically a case of hemorrhoids. Always consult your doctor to rule out other, more severe digestive disorders including IBD and colorectal cancer.

The following are other symptoms that may be noted for both types of hemorrhoids:

- Itching and irritation in the anal region
- Swelling around the anus
- Pain or discomfort
- A sensitive lump near the anus
- Leakage of feces

Treating Hemorrhoids

The majority of hemorrhoids can be treated with self-care. This care might include a sitz bath—sitting in warm water for periods of time—and applying over-the-counter ointments or creams to reduce pain and inflammation. Ensuring that you are eating a high-fiber diet and drinking plenty of water may keep internal hemorrhoids from bleeding.

Occasionally, straining can push an internal hemorrhoid through the anal opening. A doctor can often push this protruding, or prolapsed, hemorrhoid back in, but in some instances, the problem may require minor surgery. External hemorrhoids can sometimes form blood clots, resulting in severe pain, swelling, and inflammation. These can often be addressed in the doctor's office with a small incision to provide immediate relief, followed with sitz baths and medication.

For particularly stubborn hemorrhoids that do not respond to conservative treatment, a procedure known as rubber band ligation may be performed. The procedure cuts off the blood supply to the hemorrhoid with a rubber band tightly wrapped around the base of the hemorrhoid. Although this treatment is often painful, the results are usually successful. Infrared coagulation (IRC), a less painful procedure, is another treatment option that causes the hemorrhoid to harden and shrivel from exposure to laser or heat.

Anal Fissures

Sometimes initially confused with a hemorrhoid, an anal fissure is a tear or crack in the anal canal that can result in bleeding similar to that of hemorrhoids, but it is usually accompanied by intense pain and burning. Often seen in patients with CD, fissures can also be common in infants and the elderly.

Anal fissures are generally caused by constipation and straining to pass particularly hard or large stool. These fissures can also be the result of an abnormality of the anal sphincter in which you are unable to relax the sphincter enough to allow easy passage of stool. In essence, the intensely strong and contracted sphincter muscles literally tear open the anal canal.

> **TUMMY TIP**
>
> Never ignore pain in the anal area. Although accompanied by embarrassing symptoms, there are numerous causes of pain in the perianal region, many of which are not serious. Your doctor can get to the "bottom" of these symptoms and provide welcome relief with simple testing and treatment.

Most anal fissures heal naturally within a few weeks of simple treatments such as sitz baths, increased fiber and water intake, and topical creams to relieve pain. Sometimes, though, surgery is required to help relax the sphincter. The most common surgical procedure for fissures is a lateral sphincteronomy in which a slit is made to weaken the sphincter muscle, allowing the fissure to heal and avoiding the possibility of a recurrence.

Appendicitis

Although more often a childhood condition, appendicitis—inflammation of the appendix—can occur at any age. Generally considered a useless organ, the appendix is a little worm-shaped pouch that hangs from the cecum, the beginning of the colon. Appendicitis is usually the result of an obstruction that causes the appendix to fill with mucus and swell. Appendicitis may also be caused by a viral or other infection in the GI tract. In both cases, bacteria can quickly create a severe infection that can lead to a medical emergency such as a rupture. A rupture could spread the infection within the abdominal cavity and cause peritonitis (see the definition earlier in the chapter) and death if not quickly treated.

GI DIDN'T KNOW!

Darwin believed that our appendix was used for digesting leaves as primates, but as we came to consume more meat in our diets, the appendix shrank to make room for the stomach, eventually becoming useless through evolution. Even today, the original function of the appendix and its present relevance is still far from resolved.

Warning Signs

Appendicitis is usually associated with a vague, crampy pain that begins at the navel and can move toward the lower-right abdomen. This shift might indicate the emergence of peritonitis, a medical emergency. The pain often increases over a period of 12 to 18 hours, becoming sharp and debilitating. The site of the pain is tender to the touch, and it is difficult to find a comfortable position when sitting or standing. Other symptoms may include the following:

- Nausea and vomiting

- Loss of appetite

- Low-grade fever

- Constipation or diarrhea

- Abdominal swelling

Once symptoms begin, it is imperative to seek medical attention quickly to avoid complications.

Because appendicitis can mimic a number of other digestive conditions such as CD, gallbladder inflammation, intestinal obstructions or perforations, and urinary system infections, your doctor will need to rule these out. A CT scan can confirm diagnosis by visualizing inflammation, but blood work, urine tests, and simple probing of the abdomen also help to determine whether appendicitis is the cause of your symptoms. Because time is of the essence, diagnosis must be made as quickly as possible.

The Appendectomy

An attack of appendicitis almost always results in an appendectomy, the removal of the appendix. Today this surgery is usually done laparoscopically, the same way that most gallbladders are removed (see Chapter 13). If there is a complication of rupture and severe spread of infection, you may need a traditional open appendectomy. Usually, you will be back to normal within a couple days and not require any further treatment, although your doctor will want to be sure that your bowel habits are on track and there is no hint of lingering pain.

The Least You Need to Know

- Diverticulosis is the condition of having diverticula, outpouchings in the colon, and is commonly seen with age. Diverticulitis is the inflammation and infection of diverticula and requires antibiotics and occasionally surgery.

- Ischemic colitis is caused by diminished blood flow to the colon and can result in inflammation or damage to the colon lining.

- Microscopic colitis is a form of inflammatory bowel disease (IBD) that can cause excessive watery diarrhea but is not considered a serious condition.

- *Clostridium difficile* colitis, a form of infectious colitis, is often seen in hospitals and after treatment with antibiotics and can be severe and sometimes hard to treat.

- Hemorrhoids are the inflammation of veins in the rectal and anal area and are common among adults, rarely requiring more than self-care. Anal fissures are cracks in the anal canal that can cause pain and bleeding and usually heal on their own but may, in rare instances, require surgery.

- Appendicitis occurs when the appendix becomes inflamed and potentially infected. Removal of the appendix is usually required to avoid serious complications.

Additional Digestive-Related Conditions

It's time to take a closer look at the other digestive team players—the pancreas, gallbladder, and liver—and discover what kinds of problems, conditions, and diseases can affect them. Why do problems with the pancreas require immediate attention? And what's the deal with your gallbladder anyway? And given all that the liver has to do, it's no surprise that quite a few things could potentially go wrong. We'll look at all this and learn how good treatment can help repair the damage in many cases.

In addition, we'll investigate the facts about food-borne digestive illnesses: how they come about, what havoc they can cause, and how to avoid them. Finally, we'll take a close look at viruses, toxins, parasites, and the ever-popular stomach flu that can creep into our lives and cause some of the most unpleasant digestive symptoms around.

The Pancreas and Gallbladder

In This Chapter

- A pancreatitis primer
- All about gallstones
- Pancreatic, gallbladder, and bile duct cancer

Although the pancreas and gallbladder are not normally considered main players on the "A-team" of digestive organs and are not usually thought of as part of the gastro-intestinal (GI) tract, they certainly warrant a "team B" designation. The pancreas and gallbladder can be critical to your overall digestive health. In fact, when problems arise with either of these two organs, the pain may be unbearable, and the impact on the digestive process may be profound.

Problems with the pancreas generally revolve around some type of blockage. The pancreatic duct system, an intricate array of tubelike structures, carries bile from the liver into the digestive tract to break down fats and remove waste. When any of these ducts becomes blocked, serious symptoms can occur. We'll look at these as well as conditions such as inflammation of the pancreas (pancreatitis) and pancreatic cancer.

Bile also plays a huge role in gallbladder issues, which we'll examine as well. Gall-stones, the most common problem of the gallbladder, can cause tremendous pain and affect the functioning of the pancreas, too. Although many people live quite well without a gallbladder, the absence of one can create other digestive problems, again relating to bile. We'll explore these issues and more in this chapter as we take a closer look at the pancreas and gallbladder, two unsung heroes of the GI team and important players for overall digestive health.

Pain in the Pancreas

For a small organ that keeps a low profile, the pancreas can be responsible for some of the worst pain known to humans. Containing the majority of digestive enzymes required by the body, its mission, in its exocrine capacity—as opposed to its endocrine responsibilities producing insulin—is to digest relentlessly by secreting these enzymes through the pancreatic duct into the small intestine. But if the enzymes can't get out because of some sort of blockage, they become trapped and literally begin "digesting" their maker, the pancreas! In the process, inflammation and sometimes liquefaction (fluid from cell death) occur with extreme levels of pain—not unlike a knife thrust in the upper abdomen with shooting pain through to the back.

GI DIDN'T KNOW!

The power of the pancreas is so intimidating that medical students include it in their top three tips for med school: 1. Eat when you can. 2. Sleep when you can. 3. Don't mess with the pancreas!

Acute vs. Chronic

Inflammation of the pancreas, called pancreatitis, comes in two different forms: acute and chronic. Although acute and chronic pancreatitis share similar symptoms, including severe abdominal pain, they are unique in occurrence and recovery.

Acute pancreatitis, as its name suggests, comes on suddenly, lasts for a relatively short time, and then goes away almost as quickly as it arrived. Chronic pancreatitis, on the other hand, does not resolve itself and may lead to persistent pain as well as the slow destruction of the pancreas over time. However, in severe cases, either can be life threatening due to serious complications such as bleeding and infection. Enzymes, toxins, and cytokines (the body's inflammation messengers) can invade the bloodstream, resulting in major organ damage (lungs, heart, and kidneys) and even death.

Cause and Effect

In the United States, the most common causes of pancreatitis are alcohol dependence and gallstone disease. In the case of alcohol, it is believed that it may increase the secretion of pancreatic proteins that do not dissolve and that ultimately block the ducts. Damage from alcohol may not appear for many years until a sudden attack occurs. If damage is done to the ducts, chronic pancreatitis can be the result.

Gallstones, in addition to causing problems with the gallbladder, can also cause pancreatitis. Small stones can travel from the gallbladder into the common bile duct and block the *ampulla of Vater.* This blockage causes digestive enzymes arriving from the pancreas to go upstream where they came from and to begin to eat away at the pancreas, creating extreme inflammation and pain. If the blockage is not resolved, serious and critical complications can arise.

DEFINITION

The **ampulla of Vater** is the duct where bile and pancreatic enzymes meet and enter the small intestine to aid digestion. The duct is named after Abraham Vater, a German anatomist who first identified it in 1720.

Pancreas divisum is a congenital defect caused by two pancreatic ducts in the embryo that fail to fuse, causing severe backup. Pancreas divisum causes pancreatitis in 10 percent of the people who have it.

In addition to alcohol and gallstones, other causes of pancreatitis include the following:

- Blockage from tumors or scarring

- Buildup of coagulated enzymes called biliary sludge, as well as tiny stones and sandlike gravel

- *Pancreas divisum*

- Narrowing of ducts from prior pancreatitis or injuries

- High cholesterol, especially triglycerides

- Viral infections

- Scorpion stings

- Certain medications

- Trauma to the abdominal region from car accidents or blows to the stomach

Some types of medications known to cause pancreatitis include diuretics, antibiotics, immunosuppressives, anti-HIV drugs, and estrogen-containing drugs.

Symptoms and Diagnosis of Pancreatitis

The hallmark symptom of acute pancreatitis is sharp abdominal pain that often radiates to the back. It can begin or worsen after eating, last a few days, and feel more intense when lying flat on your back. People experiencing acute pancreatitis usually feel quite ill as well, with symptoms including the following:

• Nausea and vomiting

• Fever and chills

• A tender and swollen abdomen

• Rapid heartbeat

In severe cases that involve infection and bleeding, symptoms may include the following:

• Fatigue and weakness

• Lightheadedness and fainting

• Irritability and confusion

• Headache

These types of symptoms are often the result of either dehydration or low blood pressure. In fact, if blood pressure is extremely low, there exists the danger of organs not receiving enough blood, and as a result the body may go into shock.

Chronic Cases

Many of the symptoms of acute pancreatitis hold true for chronic cases, although some people may not experience much pain at all. If they do, it is likely to be deep in the abdominal cavity and radiating to the back, as with acute pancreatitis, but generally quite constant. When pain subsides, it is actually a sign that the disease has progressed and that the pancreas may have ceased producing digestive enzymes. The following are long-term complications of chronic pancreatitis:

• Diabetes from an inability to produce insulin

• Weight loss and malnutrition from poor digestion

- Anemia caused by bleeding

- Higher risk for pancreatic cancer

Testing Strategies

In the case of pancreatitis, diagnostic blood tests can reveal quite a few important facts, but often time is of the essence. During an acute attack, blood contains at least three times as much *amylase* and/or *lipase* as usual. However, these levels return to normal within 72 hours, so blood must be taken during this time frame in order for the blood test to be valid. For chronic pancreatitis, elevated levels of these enzymes may only be slight, so definitive answers are often not possible. Because elevated amylase and lipase are also associated with other GI disorders, kidney disease, and even pregnancy, these conditions need to be ruled out. Glucose levels, in addition to changes in blood calcium, magnesium, sodium, potassium, and bicarbonate, help to determine severity once diagnosis occurs.

DEFINITION

Amylase and **lipase** are digestive enzymes produced by the pancreas. Amylase breaks down starch into sugar, while lipase assists in fat digestion.

If your doctor suspects pancreatitis, he or she often orders cross-sectional imaging, especially computed tomography (CT) scans, to corroborate the diagnosis and look for severity and possible complications. An endoscopic ultrasound (EUS) can look for evidence of chronic pancreatitis such as calcifications and ductal irregularities. An endoscopic retrograde cholangiopancreatography (ERCP) allows the gastroenterologist to get a good look at ducts, remove gallstones and ductal stones, and perform a biopsy as well. Unfortunately, it is an invasive procedure that can sometimes bring on an attack of pancreatitis, so it is used only in particular cases when considered necessary.

Pancreatitis Treatment

Treatment for your pancreatitis largely depends on the cause and severity of your illness. In all cases, the immediate concern is to relieve pain, prevent unnecessary complications, and keep vital body functions going. It is not unusual to have a hospital stay so that fluids can be replenished intravenously (IV) and any imbalances including nutritional ones can be addressed and corrected. Usually an order of NPO, meaning "nothing by mouth," is given for your initial treatment. All these steps give your pancreas a chance to rest and recover.

GI DIDN'T KNOW!

Hospital patients with digestive illnesses and other types of conditions often receive the medical instruction of NPO. This term, meaning that oral food and fluids should be withheld, comes from the Latin phrase *nil per os,* literally translated as "nothing through the mouth."

Mild Cases

When the degree of your pancreatitis is mild, meaning a general lack of complications, your hospital stay is likely to be brief. As mentioned previously, fluids and nutrition are administered through an IV for a few days. If vomiting and distention of the abdominal area is a problem that cannot be stopped, a tube may be placed through the nose into the stomach to remove air and fluid that have built up.

Once you are discharged, your doctor may put you on a low-fat diet (see Chapter 17) for up to four weeks to lessen the burden on your pancreas. Supplemental pancreatic enzymes may also be prescribed with meals to help with digestion and correct any malabsorption issues. If gallstones have caused the pancreatitis, surgery to remove them or the gallbladder itself will probably take place within a week. Once this is done and inflammation has disappeared, the pancreas usually returns to normal.

Severe Cases

A great deal more time and extensive treatment is required if your pancreatitis is severe and has possible complications. If the gut cannot be fed using a tube through the nose, a process called total parenteral nutrition (TPN) may be necessary in which IV feeding is given for three to six weeks. TPN may be particularly prudent if the digestive system has been "stunned" or shut down and there is notable weight loss. In cases where pancreatic tissue has died and liquefied, forming an infectious soup-like fluid, an extremely strong antibiotic may be administered for two weeks and no longer—complications with the blood can arise beyond this point. It is also possible that this situation calls for surgery in order to remove damaged parts of the pancreas. If there is a pancreatic *pseudocyst* present (or a collection of them) large enough to disrupt the healing process, liquid needs to be drained either surgically (by an endoscopy) or by a drain through the skin.

> **DEFINITION**
>
> A **pseudocyst** is a collection of inflammatory fluid that the body walls off. Although it resembles a cyst in appearance, it is technically not a true cyst because it lacks tissue cells, thus the "pseudo" designation.

If severe pancreatitis is caused by a gallstone blockage, surgery to remove it may need to be delayed for a month or more. However, if the gallstone is still present in the bile duct and is caught early enough, an ERCP is often ordered to remove the stone. In very severe cases, it's possible to require intensive care unit (ICU) stays off and on over the course of several months. These extreme types of pancreatitis can be very dangerous, and unfortunately, recovery may not even be possible.

Chronic pancreatitis can result in lifelong pain and continued problems with digestion because of the lack of pancreatic enzymes. Physicians worry about severe cases such as these because of the possibility of unacceptable weight loss, the potential for the development of pancreatic cancer, and a dependence on potent narcotic drugs.

Living with Pancreatitis

In many cases, it is possible to have a healthy future after pancreatitis. Certain guidelines need to be followed, including dietary recommendations. They include the following:

- Ceasing all alcohol consumption, especially if this is the cause
- Following a low-fat, high-carbohydrate diet
- Managing pain with appropriate medications
- Controlling blood sugar with insulin
- Supplementing with pancreatic enzymes

Cancer of the Pancreas

Often called the "silent killer," pancreatic cancer is the fifth-leading cause of cancer death in the United States. Because it is difficult to detect early, treatment is often ineffective and survival rates are low. The majority of pancreatic cancers—nearly 95 percent—are adenocarcinomas, meaning they originate in glandular tissue, and usually involve the pancreatic ducts. It isn't until the cancer grows that symptoms associated with it begin to appear. These symptoms include those on the next page.

- Pain in the upper abdomen and upper back

- Jaundice

- Nausea and vomiting

- Weakness

- Loss of appetite and weight loss

GI DIDN'T KNOW!

Although concrete symptoms of pancreatic cancer often come later in the disease, interestingly, one of the first vague signs may be depression.

The type of jaundice associated with pancreatic cancer is sometimes referred to as "painless jaundice" because it shows typical physical signs of jaundice—yellowing of eyes and skin—but lacks any abdominal discomfort or pain. This can be a significant clue that a bile duct obstruction caused by a tumor in the "head" of the pancreas may be present. This type of cancer, when discovered relatively early and without vital blood vessel involvement, can be cured through a type of surgery called a *Whipple procedure.*

DEFINITION

The **Whipple procedure** for pancreatic cancer involves the removal of the head of the pancreas; the entire gallbladder; and parts of the small intestine, bile duct, and stomach. Then a rerouting of the digestive tract is performed by joining up remaining areas. Also called a pancreaticoduodenectomy, this procedure is named after the American surgeon Allen Oldfather Whipple who perfected it in 1935. It is one of the longest surgeries in modern medicine, taking up to 14 hours.

Risks and Diagnosis

Pancreatic cancer is most prevalent in men over 60 years of age and those who are of African American descent. However, other factors appear to increase your risk as well, including the following:

- Chronic pancreatitis

- Diabetes

- Family history

- *H. pylori* infection

- Obesity

- Cigarette smoking

- Diets high in red meat and low in fruits and vegetables

- Periodontal disease

GULP!

Although excessive and prolonged alcohol intake has been implicated in chronic pancreatitis and is therefore an indirect risk factor for pancreatic cancer, there is no proven direct link between the two. In general, however, most studies indicate a slightly increased risk for cancer of the pancreas in those who drink heavily (four or more drinks per day).

Diagnosing pancreatic cancer may initially involve blood, urine, and stool testing to check for bilirubin levels and other enzymes. When the common bile duct is blocked, bilirubin, a reddish-yellow pigment in bile made from the breakdown of red blood cells, cannot pass normally from the liver to the gallbladder to the intestine and ultimately be eliminated. Because it must go somewhere, high levels of bilirubin often appear in the blood, stool, and urine and could be an indicator of pancreatic cancer. However, other diseases also display this elevation, so further testing is necessary. Similarly, a substance known as CA19-9 is often released into the bloodstream when pancreatic tumors are present, but testing for this substance is usually done more for staging and prognosis.

GI DIDN'T KNOW!

A rare and less aggressive type of pancreatic cancer known as islet cell carcinoma involves the endocrine system. Steve Jobs, founder of Apple, Inc., underwent a successful Whipple procedure for this cancer in 2004, followed by a liver transplant in 2009.

Imaging tests provide a better chance of detecting cancer, and usually a CT scan, EUS, and perhaps an ERCP (see the preceding section) may be performed to view the pancreas as well as to perform a biopsy. Tissue for biopsy can also be obtained by using a fine-needle aspiration technique in which the doctor uses a CT scan, x-ray, or ultrasound as a guide to insert a needle into the pancreas through the abdomen.

Usual Treatment

The usual treatment options for cancer of the pancreas are surgery, chemotherapy, and/or radiation. Depending on the patient's overall health, as well as the stage of the disease and the location and size of the tumor, all or part of the pancreas may be removed. A pancreatectomy (removal of the entire pancreas) most likely also involves partial removal of other digestive organs as in the Whipple procedure, but it may also include the spleen and nearby lymph nodes. If blockage is still present, it is possible to construct a type of bypass for digestive fluids that relieves pain and jaundice. It is also possible using ERCP to insert a stent where the blockage is located, avoiding extensive surgery. Although this is not a cure, it may make the final stages of the cancer more comfortable.

Gallstone Disease

We've seen in our discussion of pancreatic conditions that the gallbladder and its function are closely related to the pancreas in a particular part of the digestive process. Both release digestive juices—bile and/or enzymes—through a duct system into the upper portion of the small intestine. Clearly, when something goes wrong with one of these organs, it is quite possible to affect the other. For example, gallstones that become lodged in the common bile duct can cause acute pancreatitis due to a backup of digestive enzymes. However, gallstones that are restricted to the gallbladder can wreak havoc as well.

GI DIDN'T KNOW!

In some cultures such as China, gallstones are collected from oxen, water buffalo, and pigs and are then dried and ground into a powder to create a pill. These pills are believed to reduce fever as well as cure internal abscesses.

Stone Formation

Gallstones fall into one of two categories: cholesterol stones or pigment stones. In America, gallstones tend to be of the cholesterol type, while in Asia, for instance, pigment stones are more prevalent. Generally speaking, gallstones can be almost microscopic in size or as large as a golf ball. The gallbladder may develop hundreds of little stones or just a single great big one. Smaller stones tend to travel and are usually the ones responsible for blockages, while larger stones often just stay where they are.

It is believed that cholesterol stones form when liquid bile contains the wrong proportion of cholesterol, salts, or bilirubin or because the gallbladder doesn't empty the way it should. These types of stones are usually quite hard and are a yellow-green hue. Pigment stones, on the other hand, are composed of bilirubin and calcium, are normally smaller than cholesterol stones, and are black or brown in color. Some highly calcified stones can actually be seen on x-rays, and some stones are actually a mixture of the two types. In addition, a sludgelike secretion of the gallbladder, often a precursor to stone formation, can resemble stonelike crystals in imaging and cause many of the same symptoms that regular gallstones may produce.

Who Gets Gallstones?

Twice as many women as men appear to develop gallstones, and most of them are middle-aged and overweight. Gender seems to play a role because of elevated estrogen production. Pregnancy, hormone replacement therapy, and birth control pills all increase cholesterol levels in bile while at the same time decreasing gallbladder emptying. Excess weight is a factor because it also results in more bile cholesterol and less gallbladder movement. The following are other factors that can contribute to gallstone formation:

- Rapid weight loss
- Fasting
- Native American heritage
- Cholesterol-lowering drugs
- Low caffeine consumption
- Lack of exercise
- High triglycerides

People who suffer from conditions that result in a high red blood cell turnover, such as anemia, sickle-cell disease, or liver dysfunction, to name a few, may also be susceptible to gallstone formation, particularly pigment stones.

TUMMY TIP

If you are a member of the "four-F" club, you are the ideal candidate for gallstones. The four "Fs" are female, fat, forty (or over), and fertile (premenopausal). Although you can't change who you are, losing excess weight may reduce your risk.

Gallstone Symptoms

"Silent stones" that do not cause pain, inflammation, or problems with the liver or pancreas are actually quite common. Many people with gallstones live completely symptom free, and stones may be discovered only during diagnostic tests for other conditions. These are generally not removed unless the patient is diabetic. However, gallstones can act up at any time, and when they do, the symptoms are usually pretty noticeable. They include the following:

- Rapidly increasing pain in the right-upper abdomen

- Pain in the back or under the right shoulder

- Nausea and vomiting

- Bloating, belching, and gas

Severe gallbladder attacks can sometimes resemble a heart attack, so quick medical attention is important, and a proper diagnosis is essential. Often these attacks come on after a particularly fat-laden meal and may begin with indigestion and abdominal discomfort, rising in pain level and lasting anywhere from 30 minutes to several hours.

A gallbladder attack brought on by an acute blockage of bile ducts is an urgent situation. If symptoms such as sweating, fever, chills, jaundice, and a knifelike pain in the back are present, *cholecystitis*, *cholangitis*, or pancreatitis may have developed, requiring immediate attention by a physician and even an emergency room visit. In fact, any suspicion of gallbladder disease should receive immediate medical attention.

> **DEFINITION**
>
> **Cholecystitis** is inflammation of the gallbladder, often caused by a duct blockage that leads to severe infection. It can be acute or chronic. **Cholangitis** is inflammation of the bile duct. It is potentially deadly, and is a medical emergency requiring immediate attention.

Detection and Treatment

By far, the best test for gallstone detection is the ultrasound. It is able to find up to 90 percent of stones and can also provide evidence of any thickening of the gallbladder wall and the presence of inflammation. Bile ducts can also be seen in relation to the positioning of any gallstones. Other types of tests may be performed if there is a suspicion of complications or infection. An EUS is more precise, while a HIDA scan (see Chapter 4) can detect acute and chronic cholecystitis.

Once a diagnosis is made, your doctor recommends the appropriate treatment. Every year, more than half a million Americans opt to have their gallbladders removed to eliminate the possibility of further painful attacks. This procedure is called a cholecystectomy and is done by laparoscopic surgery. Years ago, gallbladder removal required major surgery followed by a pretty long recovery period. The only way to get at the gallbladder was through an incision in the abdomen that cut through the stomach muscles. Today, thanks to the far less invasive laparoscopic technique, only a few small incisions need to be made in the abdominal area to allow for the insertion of a camera and tools. While watching a video monitor, the surgeon uses these tools to carefully separate the gallbladder from the liver and ducts and then removes the gallbladder through one of the small incisions. In general, a one-night stay in the hospital is all that is required, followed by a brief recovery of several days at home. During this time you are asked to refrain from activities, including lifting and stretching.

In about 5 percent of cases, traditional open abdominal surgery may be needed because of infection or other complications, particularly those involving bile ducts. Injured bile ducts left untreated can cause leakage and lead to a dangerous infection, extreme pain, and even death. Impacted stones require more intensive surgery as well and possibly an ERCP after initial surgery. In these instances, a longer hospital stay (up to a week) may be necessary, and several weeks at home with restricted activity as well as diet changes and thorough follow-up are required.

GULP!

Sometimes a gallstone—either newly created or an old one left behind—is found in a duct after the gallbladder has been removed. Weeks, months, or even years could pass before it is diagnosed, at which time it, too, would need to be removed.

Finally, it is sometimes possible to avoid gallbladder removal by dissolving gallstones. They need to be quite small and uncalcified (not hardened by calcium salt buildup), and your gallbladder must be functioning well and free of complications. This treatment involves taking a type of bile salt for several months that dissolves the bile cholesterol. Routine monitoring with ultrasound indicates progress. Appropriate for those who cannot tolerate surgery, this treatment has drawbacks as well. Diarrhea is a typical side effect, and there is no guarantee that gallstones will not reform once the medication is stopped.

Gallbladder Inflammation

Inflammation and infection of the gallbladder usually happens with gallstones, but some types of cholecystitis occur without stones being present at all. Classic symptoms include upper-right abdominal pain, fever, and elevated white blood cells. Nausea and vomiting are also common symptoms. A careful diagnosis must be made, however, because many other conditions can cause similar symptoms, such as the following:

- Peptic ulcers
- Pancreatitis
- Hepatitis
- Appendicitis
- Kidney stones

A doctor can often feel an enlarged and tender gallbladder through the abdominal wall. He or she checks for *Murphy's sign* during a physical exam, as well as for increased heart rate and breathing. These symptoms, along with blood work and an ultrasound, help with diagnosis.

DEFINITION

Murphy's sign is a simple test in which pressure applied to the upper-right abdomen causes the patient to stop breathing because of increased pain. The test is used to diagnose gallbladder inflammation but tends not to be accurate in elderly patients. Murphy's sign is named after nineteenth-century physician John Benjamin Murphy, who first described it.

From Acute to Chronic

Chronic cholecystitis is usually the result of repeated acute attacks. The wall of the gallbladder thickens, and the organ itself shrinks, losing its ability to do its job: concentrating, storing, and releasing bile. Removal of the gallbladder is the usual recommended treatment. On occasion, your doctor may consider other treatment before removing the gallbladder because people with chronic cholecystitis sometimes continue to have abdominal pain even after the gallbladder is removed.

Acute cholecystitis, more sudden and generally more painful, requires antibiotics once an infection is detected and identified. A hospital stay is mandatory, and all normal eating must cease. Once the condition is stabilized, surgery to remove the gallbladder takes place. ERCP (discussed earlier in the chapter) may be used to enlarge the common bile duct and extend the size of the biliary valve, which regulates the flow of bile and pancreatic juices into the upper small intestine. This procedure creates a new path for bile flow.

Stone-Free Cholecystitis

The most common gallbladder inflammatory condition that occurs in the absence of gallstones is acalculous cholecystitis. Between 5 and 10 percent of acute cholecystitis cases are of this more serious type and can occur after the following:

- Major surgery

- Serious injuries, burns, and infections

- Prolonged intravenous feeding

- Prolonged fasting

- Immune system deficiencies

Unlike other forms of cholecystitis, the acalculous type may be seen in children after viral or other types of infections.

The exact causes of acalculous cholecystitis are not known but may involve a problem with the gallbladder that results in obstruction of the cystic duct (the duct connecting the common bile duct with the gallbladder), and the inability of the gallbladder to contract. An ultrasound can sometimes detect this condition (although a HIDA scan is most accurate), and removal of the gallbladder typically follows.

Another type of inflammation that can occur without gallstones is called a biliary dyskinesia. This inflammation results in steady pain in the upper-right abdominal area. Abnormal gallbladder emptying may be the problem. If not, there may be a dysfunction with the sphincter of Oddi, a valve that controls the flow of digestive juices through the ampulla of Vater (see the definition earlier in this chapter) into the upper small intestine. This type of cholecystitis is sometimes associated with acute pancreatitis and is treated with medication or surgery.

Gallbladder-Free Living

The majority of people who have their gallbladders removed go on to live quite comfortably and symptom free. Some people, however, can experience something known as postcholecystectomy pain (PCS), in which continued or recurring pain is felt. Again, a sphincter of Oddi dysfunction may be to blame or internal scar tissue formation that sometimes occurs after surgery.

After a cholecystectomy, the liver continues with its bile-making responsibilities even though the gallbladder is no longer available for storage. Normally this situation does not present a problem. Sometimes, however, a continual leakage of bile causes a condition called bile acid diarrhea. The small intestine becomes overwhelmed with the amount of bile salts it receives and cannot absorb them all. Consequently, the excess spills into the colon where it has a laxative effect, causing diarrhea. Often this condition is felt as an urgency shortly after eating or even during a meal. A medication called cholestyramine usually remedies this problem, but it can decrease the effectiveness of many drugs as well as interfere with vitamin absorption. The use of fiber supplements as an alternative has been known to help some people with this particular condition.

Gallbladder and Bile Duct Cancer

Cancer of the bile ducts or the gallbladder is not common. However, women tend to develop these types of cancer more than men, and people with gallstones are also more susceptible. Many of the symptoms are similar to symptoms of gallstones and pancreatic cancer. In early stages, however, a lack of symptoms may often be the case. In general, gallbladder and bile duct cancers are discovered incidentally when things such as jaundice, unexplained weight loss, and abdominal pain are present, prompting your doctor to test for other conditions.

The Porcelain Effect and Other Risks

Sometimes the gallbladder can have the look of porcelain with a blue discoloration and brittle-looking composition. Extensive calcium content causes this condition, and it is often associated with gallstones. However, some believe that "porcelain gallbladder" puts patients at a high risk of gallbladder cancer, so when x-rays or other diagnostic tests detect the porcelain effect, doctors usually recommend removal of the gallbladder.

Other risks for gallbladder cancer are the presence of polyps—especially large ones—as well as being overweight. Certain types of cysts commonly found in people of Japanese descent can increase the risk of bile duct cancer. A condition called *sclerosing cholangitis* increases your lifetime risk of bile duct cancer dramatically as well. Ulcerative colitis (UC), Crohn's disease (CD), smoking, and certain types of parasites may also put you at higher risk.

DEFINITION

Sclerosing cholangitis is a chronic liver disease caused by inflammation and scarring of the bile ducts, which can lead to cirrhosis (irreversible scarring of the liver) and eventually liver failure.

Diagnosis and Treatment

Once your doctor suspects gallbladder or bile duct cancer, he or she is likely to order an EUS or CT scan with a needle biopsy, although an MRI can provide more information in some cases and may be requested instead. If cancer is found, further tests determine whether it has spread to the liver, stomach, pancreas, intestine, or lymph nodes. If the disease is caught early, removal of the gallbladder can be highly effective. However, if a tumor is blocking bile ducts, more extensive surgery is required and will also provide relief from pain. If the cancer is in its later stages, partial removal of other organs such as the liver may be necessary. As with pancreatic cancer, survival rates are relatively low, mainly because of late detection and progression of the disease. Sometimes chemotherapy and radiation are part of a treatment plan after surgery, although gallbladder and bile duct tumors tend to be resistant to these therapies. New forms of treatment, however, are being developed every day, and there are always clinical trials in progress that can be explored when appropriate for individual cases (see Appendix B).

The Least You Need to Know

- Pancreatic problems usually involve blockages of biliary and pancreatic ducts.
- Pancreatitis usually requires hospitalization and can be acute or chronic, often brought on by gallstones or long-term alcohol abuse.
- Gallstones, both large and small, are very common, and most people experience no symptoms from them at all.

- Gallbladders with stones that cause pain, inflammation, and/or blockages are usually removed.
- Inflammation of the gallbladder can be as serious as pancreatitis.
- Bile duct, gallbladder, and pancreatic cancers are extremely difficult to cure unless caught early.

Diseases of the Liver

In This Chapter

- Learning the ABCs of hepatitis
- Processing problems with the liver
- Advanced liver disease, cirrhosis, and cancer

As we saw in Chapter 2, the liver is such an incredible multitasker it's no wonder that on occasion things go wrong. From infection to scarring to cancer, the liver is susceptible, but miraculously it is also receptive to a number of treatments. If problems are caught early, the liver's regenerative nature helps it heal itself.

Hepatitis may be the best-known liver disease, but its types and causes are often misunderstood. There are a number of different forms of hepatitis, and we'll look at most of them in detail. Other forms of liver disease involve hindered processing of certain minerals and other substances. Hemochromatosis, which results from an overload of iron, is one that we'll talk about in this chapter. Wilson's disease and fatty liver are other conditions that can result from problems in processing, and we'll look at those as well.

Most people relate liver diseases such as cirrhosis of the liver to alcoholism, and in many cases alcohol is responsible for these types of conditions. Some people, however, can develop the same diseases without ever imbibing. We'll look at why this is so and explore treatment solutions available for severe diseases of the liver, including cancer. We'll start with the ABCs of hepatitis.

An Alphabet of Hepatitis

Simply put, hepatitis is an inflammation of the liver. Most people have heard about forms of hepatitis that are viral, such as hepatitis A, B, C, and several other letters of the alphabet. However, there are numerous nonviral causes of hepatitis as well. They include the following:

- Bacterial and fungal infections
- Alcohol and other toxins
- Drugs and medications, including steroids
- Autoimmune disorders
- Fatty deposits in the liver
- Heredity
- Some herbs and herbal teas

As with other inflammatory diseases, hepatitis can be either acute or chronic. An acute bout generally lasts less than six months, while chronic hepatitis persists longer. Acute cases normally run their course after treatment, whereas chronic cases eventually damage the liver and sometimes progress to cirrhosis.

GI DIDN'T KNOW!

According to the American Medical Association, more than five million people in the United States are chronically infected with one form or another of viral hepatitis.

The Various Viruses

Most acute hepatitis cases are caused by viruses. Each virus is unique and has its own way of transmitting itself from person to person. Here's a brief primer on the alphabet of viral hepatitis:

Hepatitis A: This type can be spread through drinking water and eating food contaminated with human feces. It is normally short lived, and there is a vaccine available to prevent it—recommended when traveling to underdeveloped countries.

Hepatitis B: Sometimes referred to as serum hepatitis, this type can be spread through blood transfusions, sexual practices, and intravenous drugs. It is the most prevalent type worldwide and can lead to chronic hepatitis and cirrhosis. A vaccine can prevent it.

Hepatitis C: This is the most common type found in the United States and is generally spread through contaminated blood and needles. There is no vaccine available, and it can become chronic and lead to cirrhosis. It is one of the main reasons for liver transplants in the United States.

Hepatitis D: This type is seen only in the presence of type B and is most often found in drug users. Most cases progress to cirrhosis, but a vaccination for type B will prevent type D as well.

Hepatitis E: This type is most often found in countries with poor sanitation, and nearly all cases in the United States are among travelers returning from underdeveloped countries. There is no vaccine available, and hepatitis E can be a major problem for pregnant women.

Let's take a closer look at the symptoms, diagnosis, and treatment of the most common forms of viral hepatitis: type A, type B, and type C.

GI DIDN'T KNOW!

Although not classified as hepatitis viruses, other types of viruses can cause hepatitis as well. They are herpes viruses, including CMV, HSV, EBV, and VZV; Epstein-Barr virus (associated with mononucleosis and perhaps chronic fatigue syndrome); and yellow fever (transmitted by mosquitoes).

All About A

Hepatitis A, although a common cause of acute hepatitis, usually goes away before causing much damage to the liver and, as a rule, does not normally lead to chronic hepatitis. Restaurants with poor sanitation and developing countries where poor hygiene is prevalent are the usual sources for hepatitis A. Vaccination against hepatitis A should be considered for the following people who are at a higher risk of infection:

- Children in communities where rates of type A are high
- Anyone living with someone infected with type A
- Staff members of chronic health-care facilities

- People with chronic liver disease

- Homosexual men with multiple partners

- International travelers to type A regions

- Injection drug users

- People exposed to nonhuman primates

- Food handlers, particularly of raw shellfish

GULP!

An outbreak of hepatitis A occurred in China in 1988 and was caused by clams from a contaminated river. More than 300,000 people became infected.

Vaccines are given as two injections over a 6- to 12-month period and protect you for 10 years.

The symptoms of hepatitis A are flulike, such as fatigue, fever, vomiting, and stomach pain. Jaundice, another symptom, usually appears only once the disease has almost run its course and you are already feeling better. An enlarged liver and blood tests, along with symptoms, provide a clear diagnosis.

There is actually no specific treatment for this type of hepatitis because it normally is eliminated by the body over a period of three to four weeks. During this time, you should refrain from preparing food for others, wash your hands frequently, and if abroad, avoid consuming water, fruit, vegetables, and shellfish that could be contaminated.

All About B

Although hepatitis B is completely preventable, it remains the major cause of liver cancer in the world. In the United States, it is responsible for 10 percent of all chronic liver disease and cirrhosis cases. It is often transmitted from mother to child in Asian countries during childbirth. In the United States, unprotected sex as well as needle sharing account for the majority of cases. Other means of transmission include tattoos or body piercing using unsanitized tools and sharing a razor or toothbrush with an infected person.

The symptoms of hepatitis B are similar to those of type A. These symptoms, along with a blood test, assist in diagnosis and help to identify whether the hepatitis is acute or chronic. Once you have a diagnosis, the goal is to put the virus into a latent state to decrease liver damage and reduce the risk of cirrhosis. Antiviral medications are used over a six-month period or longer. Because this type of virus has the ability to incorporate itself in liver cells and make the progression to cancer more likely, patients are advised to be checked annually for any abnormalities. An ultrasound or MRI and blood work show whether cancerous conditions have developed.

All About C

Hepatitis C is transmitted from blood to blood. It is less associated with sexual activity than type B and is more likely to be the result of blood transfusions, drug abuse (including needle sharing and cocaine snorting), as well as mother-to-child transfer. It has been suggested that both barbers and manicurists who use unsanitized equipment may be responsible for its occurrence in developed countries as well.

GI DIDN'T KNOW!

Because hepatitis C is strictly a human disease, research and testing for a vaccine has been difficult. However, there are vaccines under development that have so far shown promising results.

There are actually six known genotypes, subtle genetic differences that impart distinct characteristics to the hepatitis C virus. More are discovered every year. Some of them are easier to treat than others. Unfortunately, the most prevalent one in the United States—genotype 1—is usually the hardest to manage. About a third of people with chronic hepatitis C eventually develop serious liver disease and cirrhosis, often requiring a liver transplant.

Surprisingly, only mild symptoms occur in the early stages of hepatitis C, if they occur at all. Here are those symptoms:

- Fatigue

- Nausea

- Tenderness in the upper-right abdomen

- Poor appetite

- Muscle and joint pain

As the disease progresses, symptoms may include the following:

- Weight loss

- Dark urine

- Abdominal swelling

- Fluid retention

Detecting this type of hepatitis can be tricky at first because changes in the blood often do not occur for up to eight weeks from the onset of symptoms. This fact and the lack of symptoms can make hepatitis C extremely difficult to diagnose in its acute stage (although a type of genetic test called PCR may be done), and often it is not until chronic hepatitis has set in that any type of treatment is begun. Once a diagnosis is confirmed, genotyping to determine which of the six forms is present will be conducted to assist with treatment decisions.

Genotype 1, the most common form of hepatitis C, normally requires a year's worth of drug therapy through shots and pills. Interferon, one of the drugs used in treatment, is often difficult to tolerate. It causes flulike symptoms early on and can create severe side effects for many people, including depression, hair loss, and extreme fatigue. Rare side effects may include the onset of diabetes, hearing problems, seizures, or thyroid issues. In as many as 15 percent of cases, treatment may need to be discontinued. For those who continue, about 50 percent go on to recover fully. Patients with other genotypes usually have high cure rates and receive drug therapy for a much shorter time.

Nonviral Forms of Hepatitis

As mentioned previously, not all forms of hepatitis are caused by viruses. Nonviral forms of hepatitis can result from a number of causes, but most commonly are drug induced, alcohol induced, or brought on by autoimmune diseases. Most people recover from nonviral hepatitis quite easily with treatment, although some develop *fulminant hepatitis* or cirrhosis, particularly those whose disease is alcohol related.

 DEFINITION

Fulminant hepatitis is defined as massive liver cell death, which can result in complete liver failure within weeks of onset. It often causes neurological changes, including altered levels of consciousness and delirium.

Toxic Hepatitis

Drug-induced and alcohol-induced nonviral hepatitis are often referred to together as toxic hepatitis. In fact, any type of substance that is potentially poisonous to the liver falls into this category. When alcohol is involved, this type of hepatitis can take years of heavy drinking to appear, although in a small number of cases only a year or less is necessary. Toxic hepatitis is often a precursor to cirrhosis, and women tend to be more susceptible to it than men.

Toxic hepatitis caused by drugs or medication is often the result of an overdose of acetaminophen, the active ingredients in drugs such as Tylenol. For this reason, you should be extremely careful to stick to the recommended dosage on the label unless you are under the care of a physician who gives other orders. Drinking alcohol along with acetaminophen can exacerbate the risk and is not wise.

Other drugs taken on a prescription basis can also cause toxic hepatitis. Some of these drugs include the following:

- Isoniazid (for tuberculosis)
- Methyldopa (for high blood pressure)
- Antibiotics such as erythromycin, chlorpromazine, and augmentin
- Oral contraceptives
- Anabolic steroids
- Statins (for high cholesterol)

TUMMY TIP

If you are taking any type of statin drug to lower your cholesterol, such as Lipitor or Zocor, be sure that your doctor is checking your liver function by performing blood work a few times a year.

In addition to prescribed and over-the-counter medications, illegal drugs—often cut with unknown toxic substances—can cause toxic hepatitis, as can certain chemicals, mushrooms, and herbs. The inhalation of certain industrial chemicals can sometimes be so toxic that a single exposure is enough to cause liver damage. Ingestion of the appropriately named deathcap mushroom can also cause toxicity almost immediately. In general, however, toxic hepatitis takes a period of time to develop from continual exposure or use of a toxic substance. The following herbs have been implicated in cases of toxic hepatitis:

- Comfrey, a perennial herb
- Jamaican bush tea
- Germander blossoms
- Jin Bu Huan, a Chinese sedative and pain reliever
- Chaparral, used traditionally by Native Americans

Many of the symptoms attributed to viral hepatitis are similar in cases of toxic hepatitis, but it is also possible to have no symptoms at all. Sometimes only a slight elevation in liver enzymes noted on a blood work lab report is the only clue. In such a case, you and your doctor need to evaluate your exposure to and use of drugs, alcohol, and other toxic substances to attempt to identify the cause. In some cases, a simple liver biopsy may confirm the diagnosis.

> **GULP!**
>
> The U.S. government has identified 20 industrial chemicals that can cause acute liver damage or death and more than 150 others that may cause toxic hepatitis. The most common ones are the dry cleaning solvent carbon tetrachloride, the industrial chemical trichloroethylene, and the herbicide paraquat.

Once exposure to the toxic substance stops, this type of hepatitis normally subsides within days or weeks. If symptoms are particularly severe, a brief hospital stay may be necessary to provide intravenous fluids and medications to relieve nausea and vomiting and to avoid dehydration. For some, liver damage may be so severe that a transplant may be the only option.

When the cause is an overdose of acetaminophen, there is an antidote that, if administered within 24 hours, can be highly effective. Acting as a formidable anti-oxidant, the liquid antidote known as N-Acetyl Cysteine—ingested or administered intravenously—binds together the toxins so they can be excreted from the body.

Autoimmune Hepatitis

Nonviral hepatitis happens when the body's own immune system begins to attack liver cells, causing inflammation. About 70 percent of cases are seen in women between the ages of 15 and 40, and it is believed that there is a genetic component involved. Interestingly, however, when this type of hepatitis affects much older people, it is men who appear to be more susceptible than women. People of northern European descent seem to be at greater risk than other ethnicities.

Autoimmune hepatitis has the potential to be quite serious and can become chronic, leading to cirrhosis and liver failure if not treated. It may coexist with other liver diseases such as viral hepatitis and be triggered by a viral infection such as acute hepatitis A, hepatitis B, or the measles. The use of a specific form of tetracycline prescribed for the treatment of acne may also trigger this response.

Fatigue is the most common symptom of autoimmune hepatitis, although irregular periods for women and new acne breakouts may appear. As with other types of hepatitis, it is possible to experience a lack of any symptoms, especially in the beginning. When symptoms appear, they are quite similar to viral and toxic hepatitis conditions, so these must be ruled out as part of the diagnosis. Blood tests for liver enzymes will reveal a particular pattern associated with this type of hepatitis. Tests for antibodies may also shed light, as can a liver biopsy.

Early treatment has been shown not only to halt the disease but in some instances to reverse some of the damage. Treatment usually includes medications to control the autoimmune response. Prednisone, a *corticosteroid*, is often combined with other drugs. This form of therapy may be required for a year or two or may be used off and on for several years. As with toxic hepatitis, a brief hospital stay may be necessary for intravenous fluids and medication to relieve nausea and vomiting and to prevent dehydration.

DEFINITION

Corticosteroid medications are a class of drugs similar to natural hormones produced by the body and are used to reduce inflammation and treat autoimmune disorders, among other uses. They have notable side effects including increased appetite, water retention, susceptibility to infection, weak bones, and mood changes.

Metabolic Liver Diseases

The liver spends much of its time processing, storing, and eliminating substances that you take into your body either through ingestion, breathing, or directly through the skin. Drugs and medications need to be broken down into a form that you can use, while vitamins, minerals, and sugars may be stored for future use. The *metabolism* of fats from the food we eat is another big job. Occasionally, because of a hereditary defect or other condition, the liver may have problems, resulting in a buildup of certain substances that, if not treated, could lead to serious illness and disease.

DEFINITION

Metabolism is the process of breaking down or building up substances in living organisms. The term usually refers to the breakdown and transformation of food into energy.

Iron Overload

Hemochromatosis, primarily a hereditary disease, can cause iron overload in the body. Normally we retain about 10 percent of the iron in the food we eat, but people with this condition retain much more. This excess is then stored in organs such as the liver, heart, and pancreas, where it can do damage and lead to life-threatening illnesses such as cancer, heart problems, and of course, liver disease.

The genetic form of the disorder is present at birth, but it may take a few decades before symptoms appear. In order to inherit this disorder, both parents must contribute a defective gene, although you can be a carrier for hemochromatosis if only one parent has passed on this abnormality. Caucasians of northern European background tend to be more susceptible, and men are afflicted more often than women, probably because women release iron during menstrual periods.

TUMMY TIP

If a close relative has been diagnosed with hemochromatosis, it is usually recommended that you be periodically tested before serious symptoms appear.

Symptoms of hemochromatosis normally begin to appear in men between the ages of 30 and 50 and in women over the age of 50. Early stage indicators include the following symptoms:

- Arthritis, especially in the hands
- Chronic fatigue
- Low libido or impotence
- Abdominal pain
- High blood-sugar levels
- Low thyroid function

Once the disease becomes advanced, there may already be liver damage including cirrhosis, liver failure or cancer, diabetes, and cardiac issues. A bronze discoloration of the skin may also occur. Because hemochromatosis is considered rare, many doctors do not think to test for it and instead focus on the symptoms that appear. Simple blood tests, however, can determine how much iron is being stored in the body, so these should be conducted if you are at risk. Once iron levels are established, your doctor may order a special blood test to detect the gene mutation as well as a liver biopsy.

Although it sounds primitive, treatment for hemochromatosis involves the removal of blood in order to decrease iron levels. This procedure is called phlebotomy and may initially be performed once or twice a week for several months or longer while blood tests ensure that iron levels are getting lower. Generally a pint of blood is taken each time. Once iron levels are back to normal, they should be monitored regularly, and maintenance therapy of blood removal will probably take place every few months for life.

Copper Overload

Another metabolic liver disease that can cause an overload of a mineral—in this case, copper—is known as Wilson's disease. As in hemochromatosis, the liver is unable to excrete any excess into the bile and a buildup occurs. Eventually, the liver ends up releasing this surplus of copper into the bloodstream, where it circulates throughout the body and causes damage to the kidneys, brain, and eyes. Left untreated, Wilson's disease can be fatal, but if caught early most people are able to have a completely normal life.

Again, a defective gene must be provided by both parents in order for the disease to occur, and you can be a carrier with one of these genes present. As with hemochromatosis, people with immediate family members who have Wilson's disease should be checked periodically for elevated copper levels.

Symptoms generally appear in younger individuals between the ages of 6 and 20, but they can also begin as late as 40. Because this disease affects not only the liver but the central nervous system as well, it is often hard to detect because of the variety of potential symptoms that might appear. There are, however, several symptoms that when put together can shed more light than when noted individually. They include the indicators on the next page.

- *Kayser-Fleischer ring*

- Liver disease problems including jaundice

- Neurological problems such as tremors and spasms

- Personality changes and behavioral problems

DEFINITION

Kayser-Fleischer ring is the most characteristic sign of Wilson's disease. It appears as a greenish brown ring of copper deposits around the cornea of the eye and can be seen during an eye exam with a high-intensity light and microscope.

Advanced symptoms associated with cirrhosis, such as abdominal swelling and an enlarged liver and spleen, can usually be detected quite readily by your doctor. Blood and urine tests as well as a liver biopsy help to confirm diagnosis.

Treating Wilson's disease necessitates lifelong drug therapy to remove excess copper from the body. These steps stop the intestines from absorbing copper and assist the body in eliminating it. Often a low-copper diet and supplements of vitamin B_6 are recommended as well. Once treatment begins, many of the symptoms associated with this disease subside, but if scarring of the liver has already taken place, it will not be reversible. In addition, some psychological and neurological problems may take a longer time to resolve and in some cases may never be completely reversed.

Fat Overload

A condition known as fatty liver, also called steatosis, usually occurs for one of two reasons: alcoholism or obesity. It has become an increasing cause of cirrhosis of the liver in the United States and in nonalcoholics. It is also associated with metabolic syndrome, the nearly epidemic condition of having diabetes, obesity, high blood pressure, and high cholesterol simultaneously. Excess fat in the liver can damage liver cells and result in scar tissue formation—the beginning of cirrhosis. Diagnosing fatty liver early can be significant in reducing the progression to serious liver disease.

Because symptoms are relatively rare at the beginning, fatty liver may be discovered during a routine physical exam when an enlarged liver may be noted by your doctor and you feel pain or tenderness in the upper-right abdomen. Blood tests indicate a rise in certain liver enzymes and assist in a diagnosis. An ultrasound or computed tomography (CT) scan can reveal fat in the liver as well, while a liver biopsy will confirm it. In some people the liver can become inflamed, a condition called non-alcoholic steatohepatitis (NASH), potentially leading to liver failure.

GULP!

A rare form of fatty liver can occur in late pregnancy and may result in jaundice and liver failure. Treatment usually involves delivering the baby whenever possible. Acute fatty liver during pregnancy has a known genetic cause, usually present in the baby and not the mom.

More women than men appear to develop fatty liver, but no specific ethnicity seems to be at greater risk. Once diagnosed, removing the cause of excess fat in the liver is the main goal. Obviously, in cases of alcoholic fatty liver drinking must cease. In cases in which obesity is the cause, a 10 to 15 percent reduction in weight is normally recommended over a 6- to 12-month period. In many cases, fatty liver can be successfully reversed.

Cirrhosis of the Liver

As you've probably noticed about many of the liver diseases in this chapter, just about all of them, if chronic or untreated, can result in cirrhosis. A cirrhotic liver is a severely damaged one in which scarring (fibrosis) has become so extensive that the liver can no longer repair itself or do its job properly. Under normal circumstances, the liver receives and processes all blood before it is dispersed throughout the body. When the liver can no longer do this, blood remains unpurified, and usual blood flow through the main portal vein becomes difficult as well. As a result, toxins remain in the body causing dangerous conditions, and smaller veins, now overwhelmed by the amount of blood flow, are susceptible to bursting. This mounting pressure creates dilated veins called varices. They are usually located in the lower esophagus and upper stomach areas. When esophageal varices burst, bleeding is extreme and often fatal.

The following are other complications of cirrhosis:

- Malnutrition

- Frequent infections

- *Portosystemic encephalopathy*

- Increased risk of liver cancer

DEFINITION

Portosystemic encephalopathy is a condition characterized by excitability, tremors, compulsive behavior, and confusion, potentially leading to complete unresponsiveness or coma. It is caused by the liver's inability to eliminate toxins.

Symptoms and Diagnosis

Unfortunately, most symptoms of cirrhosis do not appear until there is substantial liver damage, and sometimes the complications themselves provide the first hint of the disease. When symptoms arise, they usually include the following:

- Fatigue and weakness

- Loss of appetite and weight loss

- Jaundice

- Bruising and bleeding

- Fluid in the abdominal cavity

- Swelling of the feet

- Gallstones

Once cirrhosis is suspected from blood work, an enlarged or hard liver, and various symptoms, you need a CT scan, ultrasound, or laparoscope procedure to look for signs of liver scarring and disease. Ultimately, a liver biopsy provides a firm diagnosis.

Treating Cirrhosis

As with other liver diseases, identifying and eliminating the underlying cause is the first action. Avoidance of alcohol and having a healthy diet are of utmost importance. If the cirrhosis is related to hepatitis, drug treatment is administered, and when non-alcoholic fatty liver is the cause, weight loss is mandatory. Although damage to the liver at this stage cannot be reversed, treatment can definitely slow down or stop any further harm and complications. When the liver is severely damaged and complications cannot be controlled, a transplant may be the only option.

GI DIDN'T KNOW!

The United Network for Organ Sharing (UNOS) keeps a national waiting list for liver transplants. Ranking is decided by a model for end-stage liver disease (MELD) score based on kidney and clotting function and bilirubin levels. Blood type, body size, and degree of disease also play a role on how quickly you'll get a liver, and people with blood type O normally have a better chance.

Liver Cancer

More than 90 percent of primary liver cancer cases are the result of cirrhosis from chronic hepatitis or alcohol abuse. Secondary liver cancer cases—those that have metastasized from elsewhere—are actually more common. Here we look only at the primary type and the methods used to diagnose and treat this serious disease.

There are four main types of primary liver cancer, depending on which liver cells become cancerous. They are as follows:

- **Hepatoma:** Originating in hepatocyte cells; the most common type affecting both adults and children

- **Cholangiocarcinoma:** Originating in the bile ducts; sometimes referred to as bile duct cancer

- **Angiosarcoma or hemangiosarcoma:** Extremely rare, fast-growing, and originating in the blood vessels of the liver

- **Hepatoblastoma:** Also very rare, usually affecting children under the age of 4, but generally very treatable

Symptoms and Diagnosis

As is often the case with diseases of the liver, symptoms rarely appear early. Once they occur, there is a good chance that the cancer has already progressed. These symptoms include the following warning signs:

- Weakness and fatigue

- Loss of appetite

- Unintentional weight loss

- Abdominal pain and swelling

- Jaundice

- An enlarged liver

- Nausea and vomiting

Blood tests initially inform your doctor how the liver is functioning, while imaging tests such as a CT scan, ultrasound, or MRI detect and provide information about the tumor. A liver biopsy also is done, and an angiogram can give a good view of the blood supply to the tumor. The cancer is staged from I to IV, and unless the cancer is inoperable and/or a liver transplant is recommended, treatment will probably include several different approaches.

Treatment and Therapies

Because of the liver's ability to regenerate, a localized cancer can be cut away leaving part of the liver, provided at least 30 percent is left. When this is possible, the prognosis for many people improves to between a 20 and 35 percent five-year survival rate. In some cases, a liver transplant may be the best option.

These are treatments that directly target the tumor:

- *Cryoablation*, which freezes the tumor, causing it to die.

- *Radiofrequency ablation (RFA)*, which uses heat waves to destroy the tumor.

- *Chemotherapy* is specifically targeted with a catheter in the hepatic artery that goes to the liver.

- *Embolization*, which interrupts the blood supply to the tumor.

Other medical treatments may involve water pills like Lasix and Aldactone and yearly screens for esophageal varices and hepatomas. In some cases, surgery can be useful to remove the excess fluid.

Other new therapies are being studied all the time, and clinical trials, when appropriate to individual cases, may prove to be excellent options for treatment. The key to predicting recovery from liver cancer is directly related to the size of the tumor. Small tumors (less than 5 cm in diameter) that are surgically removed and cases resolved with transplants have an 80 percent two-year survival rate. If the tumor is large, success becomes questionable. Many people who develop liver cancer already have compromised liver function, making this disease particularly difficult to treat. However, life extension is possible with an improved quality of life after treatment.

The Least You Need to Know

- Hepatitis is inflammation of the liver, and there are several different types.
- Hepatitis A, B, and C are the most prevalent, with C the most common in the United States.
- Metabolic liver disorders can cause an overload of iron, copper, or fat in the body, resulting in serious liver problems.
- Nearly all liver disorders can progress to cirrhosis, or scarring of the liver, if left untreated.
- The primary causes of cirrhosis of the liver are alcoholism and chronic hepatitis.
- Liver cancer, if detected early, can sometimes be cured by transplant or by surgery with combined therapies.

Viral Gastroenteritis and Other Infections

In This Chapter

- Viruses that cause stomach upset
- Minimizing bacterial infections
- Avoiding parasites and toxins

Everyone at some time or another has experienced stomach or bowel upset resulting in nausea, vomiting, and diarrhea. We may blame it on something we ate that "wasn't fresh" or was "sitting around too long." Or we may believe we've caught some kind of "bug" from someone else and say we have the stomach flu or a 24-hour virus. Often without truly knowing the cause, we simply ride it out with a bit of bed rest, plenty of fluids, and some very light eating until we're back to normal and up and about once again.

These types of gastrointestinal (GI) upsets can stem from a number of sources, including viruses, bacteria, parasites, and toxins. In the United States, these upsets rarely become life threatening, but in other parts of the world they are a regular and serious danger. In fact, each year there are nearly eight million deaths worldwide, mostly infants and children, as a result of gastroenteritis, the inflammation of the stomach, small bowel, and colon. Most of these deaths are from the complications of dehydration and malnutrition. How can these types of seemingly simple "bugs" become so deadly? Shouldn't we take them a bit more seriously?

Food-borne illnesses are a growing concern in our society, which relies heavily on food preparation by others. Similarly, viral and bacterial outbreaks among groups, particularly children, have become increasingly common. In this chapter, we'll look at various types of infectious substances that can affect digestive health, learn about their symptoms, and most importantly, focus on their prevention with some advice on food handling, storage, and good hygiene habits.

Viral Infections

Many infections of the GI tract tend to be lumped together as "stomach flu" or "intestinal flu." These names are often misleading because, in reality, the conditions have nothing to do with *influenza*. Gastroenteritis is actually the proper term for the inflammation of the digestive tract that we familiarly know as "stomach flu." Although autoimmune conditions and allergies may cause gastroenteritis as well, most causes are infectious, stemming from viruses, bacteria, parasites, and toxins. These infections can result in inflammation of the stomach, small intestine, colon, and even the liver on rare occasions, causing digestive distress including nausea, vomiting, abdominal cramping, and diarrhea. Severe fatigue and a fever might develop as well.

DEFINITION

Influenza, commonly called "the flu," is an acute, highly contagious infection of the respiratory tract that commonly occurs in winter and usually appears as an epidemic, affecting many people at once. Influenza is not the same as the so-called "stomach flu," although some strains, such as H1N1, can cause digestive symptoms as well.

The Norwalk Virus

The large majority of gastroenteritis cases are caused by viruses. In 90 percent of viral cases, the norovirus, also called the Norwalk virus, is the primary culprit. It is also believed to be responsible for at least half of all food-borne illnesses in the United States. Usually transmitted by consuming food or water contaminated with feces, it can also be contracted person to person and is highly contagious. Norovirus outbreaks generally occur in closed or semiclosed communities such as hospitals, dorms, prisons, or cruise ships, where rapid transmission is possible and where often the cause can be traced to food handled by one infected person.

GI DIDN'T KNOW!

There appears to be an inherited predisposition to infection by the norovirus. People with blood type O are often more susceptible than those with types B and AB, who may be partially protected.

Once you are infected with the norovirus, it begins to multiply in the small intestine, and symptoms begin within a day or two. Fortunately, the virus usually runs its course after 24 to 60 hours, and most people bounce back without any complications.

However, the elderly, children, and people with compromised immune systems may be affected longer and should be checked for signs of dehydration and other severe symptoms such as bloody diarrhea, which could indicate a more serious health situation.

The Rotavirus

The rotavirus is the second-most-common GI virus and is the one most predominant among children. This virus is the leading cause of severe diarrhea among infants and young children and is responsible for nearly three million cases of severe gastroenteritis a year. Once contracted, however, immunity begins to build so that subsequent bouts tend to be less and less severe. As a result, adults are rarely infected by the rotavirus except in unusual circumstances.

TUMMY TIP

Since 2006, two new vaccines against rotavirus A infection in children have been available in the United States and have been shown to be safe and effective. As a result, in 2009 the World Health Organization recommended that rotavirus vaccination be included in all national immunization programs.

This virus is usually transmitted by what's called the fecal-oral route, in which particles from the infected person's feces enter the potential host's body through the mouth via hands, surfaces, and objects. Poor hygiene as well as contaminated water, food, and sewage can be the means by which the rotavirus travels. Although there are seven species of this virus, rotavirus A is responsible for 90 percent of all cases, so children who are hospitalized for severe cases of gastroenteritis are usually tested for this strain by stool examination. The symptoms of rotavirus are similar to those of norovirus except that diarrhea may persist for several more days, making dehydration a real possibility unless addressed at home with plenty of fluids or in the hospital intravenously.

Two other common viruses are often the cause of gastroenteritis: adenovirus and astrovirus. The adenovirus often affects the respiratory system as well and may cause conjunctivitis—the swelling or infection of the eyelid's inner lining. Both tend to be milder and less dehydrating than the rotavirus and norovirus and are generally found in children's daycare centers and military facilities.

Prevention Tips

Infections caused by the norovirus and rotavirus are extremely contagious. To reduce your chances of infection and/or spreading the virus to others, take the following precautions, particularly if you are in a high-risk environment or have infants and children in your care:

- Wash your hands thoroughly with soap after using the bathroom, changing diapers, and before preparing and eating food.

- Disinfect surfaces and objects that have come in contact with infected individuals.

- Properly dispose of contaminated diapers and promptly wash linens and clothing that are soiled with vomit or diarrhea.

- Do not prepare food for others for several days after recovering from infection.

- Keep infected children out of daycare and adults out of closed communities when possible.

Bleach-based cleaners are best for disinfecting surfaces and clothing, while hot water and soap are recommended for thorough hand washing—not just a quick rinse. Teach kids the importance of hygiene, particularly after bathroom visits and before eating. Routine precautions can make a big difference when viral infections are on the loose.

Bacterial Infections

Although far less common than viral infections as a cause of gastroenteritis, bacterial infections are those we most often hear about on the news, particularly in relation to food-borne illnesses. In reality, "food poisoning" can be caused by viruses, toxins, and parasites, too, but bacteria-rooted outbreaks are the ones most often identified. They are also the culprits behind most of the food recall alerts and have practically become household names in advertisements for antibacterial kitchen cleaners and household products. Let's take a close look at some of the suspects.

Salmonella

Salmonella is most often talked about in relation to raw poultry and eggs, but beef, milk, and even vegetables can become easily contaminated under certain circumstances. Usually transmitted to humans through animal feces, food handlers who do not wash their hands well after touching raw meat and poultry or after using the bathroom can also be a source of transmission. In addition, *salmonella* tends to lurk in reptiles and baby birds, so handling them as pets or at zoos should always be followed up with thorough hand washing. As a rule, reptiles, including pet turtles, should not be kept in homes with infants and small children, who are especially susceptible to bacteria.

Salmonella infection, called salmonellosis, normally takes 12 hours or more to cause symptoms, which include diarrhea, abdominal cramping, and fever. Depending on your health and the extent of the infection, salmonellosis will take four to seven days to run its course, rarely requiring treatment. However, in some cases, particularly in patients whose immune systems are not strong, *salmonella* can lead to complications including *reactive arthritis*. In rare cases, the bacteria can travel from the intestines to the blood stream and may result in death unless antibiotics and hospitalization are administered.

DEFINITION

Reactive arthritis, also known as Reiter's syndrome, is a rare condition that can follow a GI bacterial infection. Reactive arthritis is usually characterized by three symptoms: arthritis, conjunctivitis, and inflammation of the urethra.

Campylobacter

Although much less of a household name than *salmonella*, *Campylobacter* is probably the most common cause of food-borne diarrhea in the United States, affecting over two million people a year. Handling and eating raw or undercooked poultry is the primary cause of this bacterial infection when it is found in single occurrences. Outbreaks, on the other hand, are usually associated with unpasteurized milk or contaminated water. The most common strain, called *Campylobacter jejuni*, or *C. jejuni* for short, is particularly adapted to the body temperature of birds, and they may carry the bacteria but show no symptoms. It's estimated that an alarming 80 to 100 percent of poultry, including chickens, turkey, and waterfowl, carry this bacteria.

GULP!

It only takes a very small number of *Campylobacter* organisms to infect humans. The amount present in just one drop of juice from raw chicken meat can cause illness.

The symptoms of *Campylobacter* infection are similar to those of *salmonella*, but there is a greater chance of bloody diarrhea or dysentery. Dysentery is a particularly severe form of diarrhea characterized by mucus and blood in the stool and is potentially fatal if left untreated. Most cases of *Campylobacter* infections in the United States, however, are resolved within two to five days without any treatment, although increased fluid intake is always recommended. In rare cases, a condition known as Guillain-Barré syndrome involving permanent nerve damage and paralysis may occur. Inflammatory skin eruptions are also possible.

Shigella

This group of bacteria, transmitted from person to person, is a common cause of gastroenteritis in small children, mainly due to poor toilet habits and hygiene. *Shigella* can contaminate food and water as well, with specific strains being prevalent in developing countries, sometimes causing deadly epidemics. Most cases in the United States are relatively mild and do not require treatment, although in some instances antibiotics may be administered. The symptoms of *Shigella* infection are diarrhea, possibly with blood, and fever. Some people show no symptoms at all but are capable of passing the infection on to others. The *incubation period* is normally two to three days, and the infection remains in the stool and is contagious for up to two weeks. For this reason, children in daycare as well as health-care workers are usually required to be symptom free for an extended period of time before returning to normal activities.

DEFINITION

The **incubation period** of bacteria-related illnesses is the amount of time required for an infection to grow and cause symptoms. Toxins, on the other hand, do not require incubation, and symptoms can appear almost immediately.

Escherichia coli

Familiarly known as *E. coli*, this type of bacteria actually has a large number of strains, most of which are completely harmless. However, some forms of *E. coli* produce a toxin similar to *Shigella* and are referred to as shiga toxin-producing *E. coli* (STEC). Of these, the *E. coli* O157:H7, or simply O157, is the most commonly identified one and is the strain usually responsible for *E. coli* outbreaks in the United States. Often dubbed the "hamburger disease" because of its association with a 1982 outbreak, this *E. coli* strain is predominantly found on cattle farms and finds its way to our tables in the form of undercooked ground beef and unpasteurized milk and juices, as well as through cross-contamination with vegetables, notably sprouts and spinach. It has also been associated with house flies.

Symptoms of *E. coli* infection can be mild or severe and are similar to other gastro-enteritis infections. Stomach cramping, diarrhea (often bloody), and vomiting usually appear within three to four days of contact. Rarely are antibiotics used in treatment, and they may actually increase the risk of developing a life-threatening condition called *hemolytic uremic syndrome* (*HUS*), particularly in children. Fortunately, most cases of *E. coli* infection are resolved within 5 to 10 days and do not require treatment other than fluid intake to prevent dehydration. While the illness is active, however, the bacteria are highly contagious, so extraordinary attention to hygiene, particularly with children, is necessary.

DEFINITION

Hemolytic uremic syndrome (HUS) is a disease resulting in acute renal failure and anemia, usually occurring after a severe bout of diarrhea from an *E. coli* O157:H7 infection, particularly if antibiotics have been administered.

Another strain of *E. coli*, which is a non-STEC type and is usually less harmful than *E. coli* O157, is responsible for most cases of traveler's diarrhea, fondly called "Montezuma's revenge." Food and water contaminated by fecal matter is the primary cause. Each year up to 50 percent of international travelers experience diarrhea and other GI symptoms while abroad, with locations including Latin America, Africa, Asia, and the Middle East the most likely sources of infection. Wilderness travelers and backpackers at home, however, can also be at risk from drinking lake water or camping in areas with poor sanitation. A traveler's diarrhea vaccine is available, although precautions still need to be taken when consuming food and water because the vaccine does not cover all potential sources of infection. Rifaximin, a powerful antibiotic that acts only on the digestive tract, can also help to prevent GI infection while traveling. Taking probiotics can be a good idea as well.

Bacteria "Ad Nauseam"

Frankly, the number of bacteria—both good and bad—that can affect our personal GI world would require a nauseatingly long list and discussion. (Did you know there are approximately five nonillion [5×10^{30}] bacteria in the world?) Here are a few of the more notable remaining ones that could cause you digestive distress:

Listeria: Found primarily in unpasteurized dairy products and processed meats such as hotdogs, *Listeria* is especially dangerous for pregnant women, as it can cause infection to the fetus or miscarriage.

Bacillus cereus: There are two distinct types. One is associated with meat, fish, and dairy and results in diarrhea six or more hours after eating. The other is connected to foods such as fried rice that are held at less than optimal temperatures, resulting in vomiting shortly after consumption.

Staphylococcus aureus: The food-borne toxin of these well-known bacteria, familiarly known as "staph," is not destroyed by heating and is usually caused by an infected food handler or mayonnaise that is left out too long. Symptoms develop within hours and last one to two days.

Yersinia: Mainly acquired by handling or consuming raw or undercooked pork, this is in the same family that causes plague. Particularly dangerous for infants, symptoms develop after four days and last up to three weeks.

Leptospira: Water and food contaminated with animal urine are the primary sources of *Leptospira*. People who work outdoors and with wildlife are most susceptible, as are lake swimmers. Severe cases can lead to kidney or liver failure.

Clostridium difficile: Although recent studies have suggested that these bacteria may be food-borne, they are more often associated with antibiotic use in hospitals and nursing homes, where the bacteria flourish in the colon after good bacteria have been eradicated along with bad. *Clostridium difficile* can lead to severe digestive symptoms and irreparable damage to the colon.

Vibrio cholerae: These bacteria are responsible for cholera, one of the most rapidly fatal illnesses in the world. Although industrialized nations have not seen an outbreak in nearly a century, some countries, including parts of Africa, are currently experiencing outbreaks. Contaminated water and shellfish are the usual means of infection.

Vibrio vulnificus: This is a close relative of the infectious agent in cholera. These bacteria are also marine in nature and can be contracted by eating seafood, especially sushi, or by swimming in infected waters, particularly with open wounds. Those with severe liver conditions such as cirrhosis are most susceptible to the life-threatening potential.

Salmonella typhi: This strain of *salmonella* is responsible for typhoid fever, a disease that's rare today in the United States but still prevalent around the globe. Food prepared by carriers of the bacteria is the common path to infection. Vaccines are available for travelers to the developing world.

> **GI DIDN'T KNOW!**
>
> Mary Mallon was a cook who was estimated to have infected over 50 people with typhoid in the New York City area between 1900 and 1907. She was quarantined twice but denied her infection up to her death in 1938. An autopsy revealed she had live typhoid bacteria in her gallbladder, however, and she was subsequently dubbed "Typhoid Mary," the first known healthy carrier of the bacteria in modern medicine.

Prevention Tips

Although it is virtually impossible to avoid all bacterial contact, there are definite precautions you can take to minimize infection both in your home and when traveling. Enough can't be said about washing and sanitizing your hands, especially when preparing food for yourself and others. Attention to sanitization and vigilant hygiene are particularly important, however, when away from home where you have much less control over sources where bacteria can lurk: food, water, and public facilities. Here are some basic tips for preventing food-borne bacteria infection at home:

- Always wash your hands before and during food preparation.
- Keep surfaces and storage areas clean with antibacterial cleansers.
- Thoroughly wash all fresh fruits and vegetables.
- Store perishable items at appropriate temperatures.
- Cook food thoroughly, particularly beef and chicken.
- Avoid cross-contamination by keeping raw meats away from other foods and washing surfaces well after contact.

- Discard food that has been left out for more than a few hours, especially those containing mayonnaise.

- Check expiration dates and avoid unpasteurized products.

When away from home, especially abroad, you should do the following:

- Wash hands often and carry an alcohol-based hand sanitizer.

- Drink bottled water.

- Wash and peel fresh fruit and vegetables.

- Avoid less than impeccably clean dining establishments.

- Get appropriate vaccines for your destination.

TUMMY TIP

Although many viral and bacterial infections often resolve themselves, always seek medical attention if you experience symptoms that are more than brief in length and/or worsen over time, particularly if your immune system is compromised due to other illnesses or medications.

What's Bugging You?

If you think only your dog or cat can harbor intestinal parasites, think again. The human digestive tract can be a real smorgasbord for these little freeloaders that enjoy living off stool or blood in the intestinal wall. Although more prevalent in developing countries because of contaminated food and water, here in the United States we can pick up these scroungers in a variety of places including public swimming facilities, egg-infested soil, and raw or undercooked meat and fish, to name a few.

TUMMY TIP

You can get your fill of all facts regarding pathogenic microorganisms and natural toxins, food-borne or otherwise, by consulting the *Bad Bug Book,* a handbook issued by the Food and Drug Administration (FDA) in conjunction with other government agencies, including the Centers for Disease Control (CDC). Available in print and online, the *Bad Bug Book* includes recent and/or major outbreaks for bacteria, viruses, parasites, and toxins.

There are two main types of parasites that can invade both the small and large human bowels: protozoa (one-celled organisms) and helminths (worms). They normally enter the body through the fecal-oral route (see the description earlier in this chapter) but can also arrive through the skin, particularly when we are barefoot. Often we carry around these parasites without a hint of their presence, but sometimes symptoms will come and go, making it particularly difficult to suspect them as a cause of infection. As with other GI infections, typical symptoms such as gas, bloating, diarrhea, and abdominal pain may be attributed to any number of illnesses.

Single-Cell Invaders

Protozoa are microscopic organisms that can be either parasitic or free living. Just one single invader can multiply in your body and cause serious infection. Intestinal protozoa normally enter by mouth contact with hands or surfaces that have touched contaminated feces, although unsanitary water supplies, especially in underdeveloped countries, can also be a source. The most common type is *Giardia lamblia* with an estimated two million infections per year in the United States alone. A large number of these cases occur in child daycare centers and recreational swimming areas. Diarrhea is the main symptom with gas, bloating, and stomach pain occurring as well. A stool analysis is required for diagnosis, and antibiotics are normally given as treatment.

Another single-cell parasite is the cryptosporidium, commonly referred to as "crypto." Although not as prevalent as giardia, it is considered to be the main cause of protozoan infection from public drinking and recreational water facilities in the United States. Both of these types of parasites have a hard coating that protects them outside the human body when they are excreted, so they tend to be resistant to chlorine treatments. In general, antibiotics are not required to treat crypto, but attention to fluid replenishment is extremely important, particularly for infants, young children, and those with a less-than-strong immune systems such as people with the HIV virus.

Worming Around

The other type of intestinal parasite that always causes gasps of horror is the helminth, or worm. Although visions of 10-foot-long tapeworms spring to mind, helminths are generally much smaller and sometimes even microscopic. There are three main types of worms that can infect the human digestive tract: tapeworms, roundworms, and flukes. Of these, the tapeworm is the most common cause of iron deficiency anemia worldwide and can be transmitted through undercooked fish and meats as well as through contact with infected feces. Intestinal worms do not replicate as protozoa do. You can, however, ingest the larvae, which later develop and grow into adults.

GI DIDN'T KNOW!

Intestinal parasitic worms have been freeloading for eons—tapeworms have even been found in a 3,000-year-old mummy! Early papyrus writings recommend garlic, honey, and vinegar as medicinal remedies.

Intestinal parasitic worms eat what we eat and can interfere with our nutritional absorption. Tapeworms, in particular, may attach themselves to the wall of the small intestine to feed. Hard to detect, the symptoms of infestation—if they appear at all— are common digestive ones such as diarrhea and abdominal pain and cramping. In severe and prolonged cases, weight loss and nutritional deficiency related diseases can appear. In rare instances, large worms can obstruct the digestive tract.

The only sure way to know whether intestinal worms are mooching your meals is through a tested stool sample. It may be necessary to take samples over a two- to three-day period because eggs and worm segments are generally released irregularly. On occasion and if large enough, you may be able to see them yourself in your stool (yikes!). Your doctor may order a blood test as well if there is a suspicion that the infection has migrated to tissue outside the intestine, which could cause cysts and inflammation.

GULP!

Intestinal pinworms are common in children and are usually detected by the "scotch-tape test." The sticky side is adhered to the anal opening at night to capture eggs and larvae as proof. Except for annoying nighttime anal itching, pinworms do not cause digestive distress and are easily treated with over-the-counter products or antibiotics.

Fortunately, medications exist that are toxic to these parasitic invaders. They are 95 percent effective in eliminating adult worms, but eggs may still remain during the treatment period. It is possible to reinfect yourself if you are not careful, so excellent hygiene is of utmost importance. A recheck of your stool by a laboratory about one to three months after treatment will indicate if the attackers have been thwarted.

Pick Your Poison

Although viruses, bacteria, and parasites can be "toxic" to our bodies and cause digestive distress and other physical ailments, technically speaking they are not true toxins. Chemical toxins that we ingest and that bring on gastroenteritis are not infectious and do not require an incubation period. These toxins are usually produced by a plant, such as poisonous mushrooms, or by certain kinds of exotic seafood. Gastroenteritis from chemical toxicity can also occur after ingesting water or food contaminated by chemicals such as arsenic, lead, mercury, or cadmium.

Nature's Defense

Mother Nature has provided many of her offspring with natural protection. These natural toxins are present in a variety of plants to discourage grazing predators because plants cannot flee from danger. Most of these toxins are not harmful to humans, but some can cause illness and even death if ingested. Here are some naturally dangerous things:

Poisonous mushrooms: All toxic wild varieties will cause vomiting and diarrhea at the very least and should never be consumed. Even expert mushroom hunters are not infallible. The amanita phalloides variety accounts for 95 percent of all mushroom poisoning deaths.

Uncooked red kidney beans: All beans contain a toxic agent called phytohaemagglutinin (PHA), but kidney beans have the highest concentration. Most cases of toxicity occur from raw beans that were soaked overnight and not cooked. Rarely is treatment required.

GULP!

People with an inherited deficiency of the enzyme glucose-6-phosphate dehydrogenase (G6PD) that protects red blood cells should avoid fava beans because they can cause gastroenteritis, fever, anemia, and even fatal poisoning.

Nightshade plants: For centuries, members of this family including potatoes, tomatoes, and eggplant were deemed poisonous because of solanine, a natural protective toxin. Today, we know we need only avoid the foliage and green-tinged flesh of these plants to avoid digestive distress.

Rhubarb leaves: The reddish-pink stalks of this "pie plant" are a staple of summer baking, but avoid the foliage and flowers that contain high levels of toxic oxalic acid salts.

Seafaring Toxins

Marine life can harbor natural toxins as well. These toxins are present in the fish themselves from either consuming them in their diet or naturally producing them as protection from predators. They are unlike food-borne bacteria that are usually associated with poor handling or contamination of fish and shellfish. Shellfish toxins, in particular, can cause severe neurological disorders as well as digestive problems. Here are some of the most common types of bony fish food toxins.

Ciguatera: More than 400 reef fish species living in warm, tropical waters carry this toxin from eating microscopic sea organisms. Larger, older fish that are higher up the food chain such as eel, snapper, and grouper are most often affected. Cooking does not destroy the toxin, and flavor is not altered. Digestive symptoms occur within hours and are not normally treated, but neurological symptoms can last for months or years.

> **GI DIDN'T KNOW!**
>
> One type of shellfish poisoning caused by domoic acid from algae alters brain function and typically affects seabirds. A supposed 1961 outbreak near Santa Cruz, California, caused thousands of birds to become frantic and provided inspiration for Alfred Hitchcock's movie *The Birds.*

Tetrodotoxin: The pufferfish or fugu, a sushi delicacy, carries this natural poison that can be deadly to diners if the fish is not prepared correctly. Both digestive and respiratory symptoms can occur, with death a real possibility. No known antidote exists. Only specially licensed chefs can prepare and serve fugu.

Scrombroid: This poisoning is caused by a buildup of histamine as a result of decay in species such as mackerel, tuna, and mahi-mahi. Nausea and vomiting occur almost immediately after consumption, and symptoms are often mistaken for a seafood allergy. Storing caught fish properly prevents development of the toxin, while antihistamines can help treat symptoms.

Pesky Pesticides

Pesticides are designed to protect us from harmful insects, pathogens, and other disease-causing elements. The severe drawback of their use, however, is their potential to cause illness when we consume foods that have been treated with them. Mild to severe symptoms can occur, including cramping, diarrhea, and headache, and many long-term effects are yet unknown. Although the Environmental Protection Agency (EPA) monitors the amount of pesticide "residue" allowed on food before it gets to our tables, careful cleaning is still necessary. In particular, infants, children, and pets tend to be more susceptible to the effects of these toxins, so experts recommend taking certain precautions when preparing and serving food that has likely been treated with chemical toxins. Here are some important safety measures:

- Wash and scrub fresh produce under running water.
- Peel and trim fruits and vegetables when possible.
- Discard outer leaves of leafy vegetables.
- Remove skin and fat from poultry and fish.
- Consider purchasing organically grown alternatives.

The Least You Need to Know

- Viruses, bacteria, parasites, and toxins can cause gastroenteritis, the inflammation of the stomach and bowel.
- The norovirus and rotavirus are the most common types of GI viruses and are highly contagious.
- Bacterial infections are usually food-borne and can result in mild or severe GI symptoms.
- Parasites and toxins can also cause gastroenteritis.
- Most infections resolve on their own, but some may be life threatening and require immediate treatment.
- Take precautions to minimize your chances of infection and the spread of infection to others.

Maintaining Good Digestive Health

When you're feeling good, you certainly want to stay that way. But how can you be sure you're doing the best you can for your digestive system? In this final part—perhaps the most important one—you'll learn the facts not only about maintaining your digestive health, but also about continuing to improve an already healthy system. From facts about fiber and supplements to natural and alternative remedies and lifestyle recommendations, you'll be well on your way to your best digestive health yet.

We'll also assist you in making specific food substitutions and menu selections that may be necessary to keep your digestive system on the best track and to ensure that you receive all the nutrition your body requires for overall health. From lactose free to low fat, you'll be well versed in specialty eating in order to keep you at your digestive peak while feeling healthy, vigorous, and fit.

Eating and Living Well

Chapter 16

In This Chapter

- The components of a healthy diet
- Fiber, EFAs, prebiotics, and probiotics
- Lifestyle changes that improve digestive health

If everyone in the world ate a healthy diet, exercised, didn't smoke, and got regular preventive checkups, most doctors—particularly gastroenterologists—would be out of work. Although, as we've seen with many digestive health conditions and diseases, a genetic factor is often at play, our dietary and lifestyle habits often influence our risk of developing a number of gastrointestinal (GI) problems and can even increase any risk posed by our genes. If we make improvements in both diet and lifestyle, we can definitely reduce that risk and improve our chances of leading long and healthy lives.

In this chapter, we'll examine the elements of a healthy diet and how they can contribute to your digestive and overall health. We'll take a close look at different types of fats and carbohydrates to discover that they're not all bad and, in fact, can be quite beneficial. Fiber will get some well-deserved press as well, and we'll learn about the importance of prebiotics and probiotics in the digestive tract.

Lastly, we'll address the question of lifestyle and digestive health with recommendations for creating a healthy eating environment as well as breaking bad habits and getting a little exercise. By the end, you'll be well equipped with the essential information you need to eat well, live well, and improve or maintain your essential GI health.

What Is a Healthy Diet?

If you're not exactly sure what a healthy diet is, you're not alone. Thanks to the enormous amount of information Americans receive through many media outlets regarding health, it's easy to get confused. When it comes to what we should or shouldn't eat, the information can be downright perplexing. What's good for us one day is suddenly taboo the next. New studies and revised dietary recommendations appear to crop up nearly every day. Unless you're a *registered dietitian (RD)*, you probably don't have time to keep track and sort through it all, much less apply it to everyday life.

DEFINITION

A dietitian is an expert in diet and nutrition who promotes good health through proper eating. A **registered dietitian (RD)** is certified by the American Dietetic Association (ADA) after meeting strict educational and professional requirements.

If you're baffled by the basics of healthy eating, it's best to simply start at the beginning. By familiarizing yourself with the building blocks of diet and nutrition, you'll be better able to understand how the specifics can affect your overall health as well as your digestive health. So here's a quick rundown of what you need to know.

Getting Down to Basics

A healthy diet is one that helps to maintain or improve health by providing appropriate amounts of nutrients. In general, nutrients are classified as either macronutrients (needed in large quantities) or micronutrients (needed in smaller quantities). Vitamins and minerals are micronutrients, while macronutrients are familiarly known as proteins, fats, and carbohydrates. Each macronutrient provides energy in the form of calories and plays an important role in the body as well. For instance, protein is required for repair and growth, while fat is needed to form cell membranes and absorb certain micronutrients. Carbohydrates, although recently given a bad rap in the weight-loss world, contribute to a number of processes including a healthy immune system and are, in fact, the preferred energy source of the brain.

GI DIDN'T KNOW!

In addition to protein, fat, and carbohydrates, both fiber and water are technically considered macronutrients. Like vitamins and minerals, they are required by the body even though they do not provide energy in the form of calories.

Finding a Balance

When you hear people talk about eating a balanced diet, they are referring to the amounts of macronutrients we consume. Although you will no doubt run across much disagreement about appropriate proportions of protein, fat, and carbohydrates, the following is a good goal to shoot for when planning your percentage of daily calories:

- Protein: 20 to 30 percent

- Fat: Up to 30 percent

- Carbohydrates: 40 to 60 percent

Clearly, if you are dealing with a condition or disease that requires an alteration in these percentages, you'll need to heed the recommendations of your doctor and/or dietitian. In fact, in Chapter 17, we'll look at several specific diet plans you may encounter if dealing with some of the digestive disorders we discussed. For the most part, however, these guidelines are a good place to begin.

Within these percentages, it is the quality of each macronutrient that is particularly important. For example, protein derived from fish and vegetables (such as soy) is often a better bet than those from animal sources that may be particularly high in saturated fat. In fact, saturated fat should account for no more than 10 percent of your daily fat intake because it is responsible for elevating cholesterol and causing blood flow blockages, not only to the heart but to the colon as well. (See the discussion on ischemic colitis in Chapter 12.) Saturated fats include high-fat dairy products (such as cream, butter, and cheese) as well as fatty cuts of meat, all of which are all best consumed in small quantities. Most monounsaturated and polyunsaturated fats (such as those found in olive oil, nuts and their oils, fish oil, and avocados) are much better for us. And, of course, avoiding products that contain *trans fats* is particularly important. In many ways, these artificially created fats are worse than saturated fat because they can increase bad cholesterol (LDL) while decreasing the good kind (HDL).

DEFINITION

Trans fats, also called trans fatty acids, are created by turning liquid oils into partially solid ones through a process called hydrogenation. Used in many processed foods, they increase shelf life, improve taste and texture, and often reduce the need for refrigeration—but at a risk to your health.

When Fat Is Fabulous

While we're on the subject of fat, one of the best things you can do for your digestive—as well as overall—health is to increase your intake of omega-3 fatty acids. Along with omega-6 and omega-9 fatty acids, they constitute what are called the essential fatty acids (EFAs). They are essential because we must have them in order to survive. Necessary for healthy cardiovascular, immune, and nervous systems, as well as having anti-inflammatory properties, omega-3, in particular, appears to be sorely lacking in most people's diets. This deficiency may be partly responsible for many physical as well as mental diseases including depression and Alzheimer's.

Although it's possible to add essential fatty acids to your diet through supplements, eating sources of EFA, particularly fish containing omega-3, appears to have the greatest impact. These sources include salmon (especially wild salmon), sardines, herring, mackerel, bluefish, and albacore tuna. In fact, consuming two to three portions of these fish per week may be enough to make a difference in maintaining or improving health.

> **TUMMY TIP**
>
> For vegetarians and those who are not particularly fond of fish, EFAs can also be found in a number of plant sources including flaxseed, walnuts, and purslane, a popular wild green used in Hispanic cooking.

Categorizing Carbs

Not that long ago, carbohydrates were simply categorized by whether or not they were complex or refined. Common sense told us that a carbohydrate that was complex was closer to its original state than one that was refined, or processed more, and consequently was a healthier alternative. So, for example, whole grains, brown rice, and whole wheat were better for us than white bread, white rice, and puffy cereals that had been stripped of their protective bran coating and fiber—and most of their nutrition—to boot. Then, in the last decade, a method of categorization became popular that helped differentiate "healthy" carbohydrates from "not-so-healthy" ones called the glycemic index. It also ended up causing a little confusion.

The glycemic index tells us how much our blood sugar rises after eating a particular carbohydrate. On a scale of 0 to 100, with pure glucose at the top, carbohydrates are classified as low (55 or less), moderate (56 to 70), or high (greater than 70). Those carbohydrates that are rapidly digested and cause quick spikes in blood glucose are not particularly good for us because they can put stress on the pancreas, which must produce a flood of insulin in order to bring glucose levels down to normal. For diabetics in particular, who need to monitor their blood-sugar levels, high glycemic rated foods can be particularly disruptive. For all of us, quick rises and falls in blood sugar can negatively affect our moods, appetite, and weight. Armed with this limited information, diet gurus and popular weight-loss programs began labeling carbs as "good" or "bad" with some vilifying carbohydrates altogether. Unfortunately, as often happens, much of the value of the glycemic index became lost in the sensation.

TUMMY TIP

When it comes to consuming carbs, always stick to reasonable serving sizes. When eaten in moderation, no carbohydrate is off limits as part of a healthy diet.

What's particularly important to recognize is that most of the lower glycemic rated foods have something the others don't—fiber. In general, those with a higher glycemic index value were lacking in fiber. But there were exceptions to this general rule, beginning much of the confusion. Many diets shunned eating carrots, for example, because their glycemic rating was quite high. What those diets didn't mention was that you'd have to eat a couple pounds of carrots at one time for them to have such an effect on glucose (excluding other foods as well). Unless you're a rabbit, you're not likely to do so.

The truth is that we tend to eat foods in much smaller amounts in combination with other foods. This combination can dramatically affect the overall glycemic rating of an entire meal and its ultimate effect on glucose levels. Confused by terms such as "glycemic load" and "amylose content," the American public got pretty much lost before anything useful sank in, although there are several good resources in books and online that provide solid information and lists of foods (see Appendix B). In places such as Australia and Britain, the glycemic index and its nuances have come to be recognized as a valuable part of dietary considerations, and it even appears on food labeling there. Here in America, we occasionally see some diet programs in media that boast "glycemically balanced" meals, but for the most part we've yet to embrace the value of the index. If you are diabetic, learning about the glycemic index may help you control your disease which, as we've seen, can be a major risk factor for many types of GI diseases.

Why Fiber Is King

Throughout our discussions of digestive symptoms, conditions, and diseases, fiber comes up again and again. Diets low in fiber are often the cause of occasional and chronic constipation. Lack of fiber can contribute to diverticular disease, colitis, and hemorrhoids. Including more fiber in your diet can alleviate symptoms of inflammatory bowel disease (IBD), including Crohn's disease (CD), and can help with irritable bowel syndrome (IBS). Fiber also feeds a lot of those friendly bacteria in the colon that work so hard to keep us healthy. So what exactly is fiber, and how does it work its magic?

Dietary fiber, sometimes referred to as roughage, is the indigestible part of plant foods that moves through the digestive system and eases bowel movements. There are two types, *soluble fiber* and *insoluble fiber*, both of which are important to good digestive health. Both can also be present in the same food source. For example, the skin of a plum is an excellent source of insoluble fiber, while the pulp provides soluble fiber.

DEFINITION

Soluble fiber dissolves in water, bulking up and softening stool while slowing the absorption of glucose. **Insoluble fiber** does not dissolve in water, passing largely unchanged through the digestive tract, also adding bulk to stool and facilitating regularity. One recently published study showed soluble fiber to be better than insoluble fiber for people with IBS.

The American Dietetic Association (ADA) recommends that the average healthy adult should consume between 20 and 35 grams of dietary fiber a day. Most of us eat barely half this amount, often much, much less. If we want to know why we are a nation that suffers from abundant digestive disorders, this is a pretty good place to start the discussion. Remember that fiber can absorb water and expand, which is why we often feel less hungry after eating a fiber-rich meal. On the other hand, when we primarily consume low-fiber foods, we tend to continue eating, often requiring greater quantities before we feel satisfied. Unlike foods rich in fiber that can sustain us for a while, low-fiber foods cause us to get hungry again much sooner. This hunger leads to a cycle of overeating, frequent junk food snacking between meals, and ultimately taking in far more calories and fat than we need. The result, in many cases, is obesity. We've already seen how obesity can create an increased risk for many of the digestive disorders we discussed, from acid reflux disease to colon cancer.

If you are overweight or obese, losing excess pounds will definitely make a difference in your digestive and overall health now and in the future. Although there are myriad plans and diets you can follow, the simple truth is that unless you are burning more calories than you are taking in, you will not lose weight. Whatever approach you decide to try, make sure that exercise is a part of it and that sensible, slow-but-sure strategies are at its core.

Crash diets and those that completely exclude necessary macronutrients such as fat can result in the depletion of certain micronutrients. For example, vitamins A, D, E, and K are fat-soluble nutrients that require the consumption of fat in order to be absorbed. Drastic changes in diet can also put stress on the digestive system, so be wary of sensational approaches and fantastical claims. Any weight-loss diet that forbids fresh fruit, vegetables, and whole grains that are high in fiber is not healthy and will probably create more problems in the long run.

GULP!

Don't become a "serial fad dieter." People who jump from one diet to the next, especially highly restrictive diets, can develop digestive, cardiac, and emotional problems by putting stress on the body.

As part of a healthy program, fiber is essential. If you find that you can't take in all the fiber you would like strictly from food, adding a fiber supplement to your diet is certainly possible. If you suffer from any specific digestive conditions, speak with your doctor about the best fiber supplement choice for you.

Vitamins and Minerals

If you are consuming a well-balanced diet with plenty of fresh fruits and vegetables, lean protein, and wholesome grains, you are probably getting all the vitamins and minerals (micronutrients) your body requires. This isn't to say that taking a multi-vitamin and mineral supplement is a bad idea. It's not. But unless you are at risk of developing certain conditions or are suffering from a disease that naturally depletes your body of specific vitamins, taking extraordinary amounts of supplements is not advisable. Many vitamins and minerals simply cannot be stored by the body and end up literally going down the drain. Others can, in some instances, create dangerous symptoms of their own.

As we've seen with certain digestive conditions such as celiac disease, Crohn's, and ulcerative colitis (UC), anemia can be a concern due to a lack of iron or vitamin B_{12}. In these cases, your doctor will prescribe specific doses for you to take and recommend reliable sources for purchase. For most women, the risk of osteoporosis can be countered with calcium and vitamin D supplementation, particularly if their dairy intake is low. It may also be helpful for those at higher risk of developing colon cancer. If you are interested in taking vitamin supplements as a preventive measure for any disease, be sure to speak with your doctor about the recommended dose.

TUMMY TIP

Whenever you are asked to list your medications at a doctor's office or hospital, always include any vitamin, mineral, or herbal supplements you are taking on a regular basis. This information is important for your doctor to know in evaluating your symptoms and in prescribing treatment and drugs.

Unfortunately, the U.S. Food and Drug Administration (FDA) does not scrutinize supplement suppliers as carefully as it should, so sometimes you may not even be getting exactly what the label claims when you purchase various vitamin products, particularly blends that include herbs. Hopefully, future regulations will take the guesswork out of most of these purchasing problems, but until then it is pretty much "buyer beware."

Making Friends with Bacteria

"Friendly bacteria," also called probiotics, are live microorganisms that can help to protect the body from "unfriendly bacteria" that often contribute to many of our digestive problems and conditions. Although we are still examining the numerous ways and means that probiotics beneficially affect us, we know they are critical to the development and function of the immune system, which in large part is located along the lining of the digestive tract. As for their effect on specific digestive conditions and diseases, there is good evidence to suggest that probiotics can be helpful with IBS, IBD, recurrent urinary tract and yeast infections, as well as diarrhea related to antibiotic use.

GI DIDN'T KNOW!

The term *probiotics*—which literally means "for life"—was first introduced in 1953, in contrast to the term *antibiotics*—"against life"—which was coined in 1942 by Selman Waksman, who went on to isolate over 15 different antibiotics.

Recently, there has been enormous interest in prebiotics as well. These are fiber-like substances that can not only increase the numbers but also the actions of our probiotic friends, providing them with necessary food to do their jobs. Inulin, a class of fiber found typically in root vegetables, and fructooligosaccharide (FOS), found in many fruits and vegetables, are just two types of prebiotics you may have heard about. With the help of prebiotics, probiotics can more successfully compete with the trillions of harmful bacteria present in the colon as well as those that are merely useless.

Unfortunately, the delicate balance of prebiotics and probiotics in the digestive tract can be easily disrupted, especially when one is taking antibiotics for illnesses and infections. Antibiotics do not discriminate between the good guys and the bad guys, killing our friends in addition to our enemies. Antibiotics are not the only assassins: Stress, chlorinated water, anti-inflammatory drugs, chemotherapy, and alcohol can destroy the good guys in record numbers, too.

Eating live active cultures (such as those found in some yogurts) and other fermented foods (such as many soy products) can help to replenish the supply. Taking probiotic supplements can certainly help as well. However, there is some discussion as to whether stomach acid might render the probiotics we consume useless before they even have a chance to reach the colon. Current research is looking into the possibility of extracting the DNA of probiotics and developing alternate ways of introducing them to the body. Supplements of both prebiotics and probiotics called synbiotics are gaining a lot of attention as well. Still, it's not a bad idea to include both probiotic- and prebiotic-containing foods in your diet when possible, as a step toward maintaining or improving your digestive health (see Chapter 17). For a detailed, up-to-date discussion of the scientific investigation of probiotics and prebiotics, check out the International Scientific Association for Probiotics and Prebiotics (ISAPP) website (www.isapp.net).

A Word About Water

Your body requires continual replenishment of water. Depending on its size, between 55 and 78 percent of the human body is water, excreted through urine and feces, through sweating, and by exhalation of water vapor in the breath. With physical exertion and heat exposure, water loss increases and daily fluid needs may increase as well.

There has been a great deal of discussion as to exactly how much water we should drink daily. Recommendations have varied from six to eight glasses per day to nearly a gallon per day. In general, drinking noncaffeinated beverages in the amount of 2 quarts or so is, under normal circumstances, quite sufficient. If we are eating plenty of fruits and vegetables, we'll be getting water from them as well.

TUMMY TIP

When you drink alcohol or caffeinated beverages (including coffee, tea, and soda), about 1 cup of water is actually removed from your system by the diuretic effect that increases water output from the kidneys. You need 2 cups of water intake to be ahead of the game.

As we've seen, water is critical in helping to alleviate constipation, and when you are eating a good amount of fiber, more water is also necessary to assist in its movement through the digestive tract. Drinking plenty of water can also help alleviate some of the initial symptoms of gas and bloating that often result from eating fiber-rich foods when you are not accustomed to eating them. All in all, drinking plenty of water is a good idea. If you are often thirsty, your body is telling you that your water intake needs to be increased.

GULP!

In rare instances, it is possible to drink too much water, causing a condition known as hyperhydration or water intoxication. Hyperhydration occurs when the normal balance of electrolytes is not replenished along with excess water intake as a result of severe diarrhea, strenuous exercise, or so-called water drinking contests. Excess water intake can also lower sodium levels and, in extreme cases, result in confusion or seizures.

What's a Healthy Lifestyle?

Throughout this book, we've seen how many of our bad habits can put us at greater risk of developing digestive problems and diseases. From lack of exercise to over-indulgence in food and drink, we are often our own worst enemies when it comes to creating fertile ground for future problems. Although we can't suddenly become epitomes of living well overnight, there are certainly positive steps we can take toward that goal. Here are just some of the actions you can take now to maintain or improve your digestive health.

Mindful Eating

Even if you are already eating a nutritious and balanced diet, how you eat may still need improvement. Dashing off after a meal, eating on the run, and skipping meals are not the best of habits. To help your body get the maximum benefit from the foods you eat, practice these good eating habits:

- If you are alone, focus on the food, not the TV, computer, or newspaper.

- If you are with family and friends, sit down together and enjoy each other's company as well as the food.

- Take small bites, eat slowly, and chew food thoroughly.

- Don't overindulge in alcoholic beverages.

- Stop eating when you are no longer hungry, not when you are stuffed.

- Avoid eating late at night.

- Take time to relax after a meal.

GI DIDN'T KNOW!

Sitting down to dinner as a family has been shown to produce smarter kids while also reducing their likelihood of smoking, drinking, and drug use.

Daily Exercise

Regular exercise, even a brief daily walk, can make a big difference in your digestive health. Exercise brings oxygen into your digestive system and helps it do its job better. Exercise also helps move things physically through the tight turns of the digestive tract, controls appetite, and increases your metabolism so you are able to burn calories more efficiently and maintain a healthy weight.

A sedentary lifestyle is often the cause of chronic constipation. Particularly for IBS sufferers, exercise can not only help resolve digestive symptoms, it is often beneficial in alleviating stress, a large contributing factor of the symptoms themselves. Finding an activity that you enjoy is a key element in developing an exercise plan. Clearly, if you don't like what you're doing, you won't continue. Whether your exercise is swimming, bike riding, or a leisurely stroll in the park, a lifestyle that includes exercise will prove to be one of the best preventive measures you can take for digestive health.

Break Bad Habits

Smoking is, of course, one of the worst things we can do for our overall health as well as our digestive health. As we've seen, smoking can contribute to acid reflux disease, CD, and many other serious GI conditions, including cancer of the esophagus, stomach, and colon. As a known carcinogen, even secondhand smoke affects the health of those you live with and increases their risk of developing a host of conditions and diseases.

Nicotine is a highly addictive drug. In order to quit, smoking needs to be approached in the same way one might tackle an addiction to alcohol or other drugs. Speak with your doctor when you are ready to quit so that he or she can recommend or prescribe medications and tools to help you. Like tackling other addictions, smoking cessation is most successful with a strong support system. Groups, friends, and family can help you through the initial and most difficult period as well as keep you on track in your quest for a smoke-free life.

Excess alcohol consumption is another risk for numerous digestive conditions and is one of the most influential dietary factors associated with GI diseases. It can damage the digestive tract and cause chronic liver problems, as we've seen. It is also responsible for many cases of ulcers, bleeding of the stomach lining, esophageal cancer, and harm to the pancreas.

Drinking in moderation has shown some benefit to cardiac health and overall health, particularly wine consumption. But if you are not a drinker, don't start now. There are plenty of other lifestyle choices that can help you maintain good health. Much of the benefit of alcohol, which lies in its levels of healthy *polyphenols*, can be obtained in other beverages and foods. Resveratrol, one of the key antioxidants found in red wine, is also present in fruits such as grapes and pomegranates as well as in peanuts, tea, and chocolate.

DEFINITION

Polyphenols are antioxidants and a class of phytochemicals naturally present in plants. Polyphenols may protect against the damage of free radicals, molecules with unpaired electrons thought to cause tissue damage in the body.

Relieve Stress

More and more, we find that chronic stress can be a contributing cause of disease. In a hectic world, it's often difficult to find moments of relaxation or time to participate in activities that are enjoyable and stress relieving. Make a point of recognizing when stress is getting the better of you and take steps to reduce stressful circumstances as best you can. Highly stressful jobs and relationships can harm your health, including your digestion. We can't always run away from stress in our lives, but we can help to alleviate it with activities such as meditation, yoga, exercise, and a variety of therapies that teach us how to cope.

See Your Doctor

Regular preventive health visits should be part of your plan to improve or maintain digestive health. Whether for a colonoscopy screening or periodic blood work, keep yourself up-to-date with appropriate tests and exams for your age. Catching problems early will always increase your chances of recovery. Know your family history and what conditions you may be prone to developing, such as celiac disease or colon cancer, and get tested sooner rather than later.

Finally, maintain an awareness of your body and how it is functioning. There is no one who knows when something might be wrong better than you do. Unusual pains, changes in bowel habits, problems with particular foods, and general lack of energy and zest for life can often indicate that something is brewing. Keep your doctor informed of any and all symptoms you encounter during routine exams and seek medical help when sudden problems arise.

The Least You Need to Know

- A healthy diet consists of a good balance of macronutrients—protein, fat, and carbohydrates.
- A diet that includes lean protein, is low in saturated fat, and is high in fiber-rich carbohydrates is ideal.
- Adding essential fatty acids (EFAs), prebiotics, and probiotics to your diet can assist in maintaining digestive health.
- Daily exercise contributes to good digestion and overall health.
- Ending bad habits such as smoking and excess drinking reduces your risk of developing many GI diseases.
- Preventive screenings and exams are essential to maintaining good health.

Food Allergies and Specialty Diets

In This Chapter

- Food allergies versus intolerance
- Why restricted eating may be required
- Special diet plans for special circumstances

Some of us have the pleasure of being able to eat anything we want without repercussions or regrets. But many people find that certain foods are difficult for them to digest. Having an intolerance to specific types of food is not uncommon and is something that often happens as we age. Food allergies, however, are usually something we are born with, and they can create an enormous amount of stress and apprehension—sometimes even taking the joy out of eating altogether.

In this chapter, we'll look briefly at major food allergies and how to know whether you are allergic or simply intolerant. We'll also look at circumstances in which a restricted diet may be necessary because of a condition, disease, or temporary need to heal. Although conditions such as celiac disease require the strict elimination of foods containing gluten, a low-residue diet may be required only for a brief time after an acute attack of a lower gastrointestinal (GI) disorder.

Having to watch what we eat is never fun. Ask anyone who has been on a weight-loss diet! But when your digestive health or overall health is at stake, restrictions are imperative if you hope to recover successfully. Whether for a temporary period or the long haul, you'll be well acquainted with the most common GI specialty diets that may be necessary in order to keep you healthy and on track for an improved digestive future.

When Food Is Your Foe

What makes some people unable to eat nuts or dairy products without experiencing discomfort at best or a life-threatening reaction at worst? Today, allergies and intolerances to food are more common than they used to be, particularly in children. Why this is so is not clearly known, but we do know that by restricting or eliminating certain foods from our diets, we can not only feel better but avoid serious reactions or complications that might arise.

Determining whether or not you actually have an allergy to certain foods is key. If you keep a food diary, you may be able to point to specific meals that cause particular problems, something always helpful for a doctor to see. But serious food allergies can be confirmed only by a physician who specializes in this area, or an *allergist-immunologist*. If you suspect that you or a family member is allergic to, say, peanuts or shellfish, you'll be referred to these types of specialists in order to get a concrete diagnosis.

DEFINITION

An **allergist-immunologist** is a physician specially trained to manage and treat asthma and other allergic diseases and is sometimes also trained in pediatrics. In the United States, physicians who hold certification by the American Board of Allergy and Immunology (ABAI) have successfully completed an accredited educational program and an evaluation process.

Common Food Allergies

A food allergy is an adverse immune response to a food protein and is distinctly different from other adverse responses to food, such as food intolerance. Here are the most common foods to which people are allergic:

- Dairy products
- Eggs
- Peanuts
- Tree nuts
- Seafood
- Shellfish

- Soy

- Wheat

These are often referred to as "the big eight," and they account for more than 90 percent of all food allergies in the United States. However, allergies to seeds—particularly sesame—are increasing and are sometimes included in this list.

GI DIDN'T KNOW!

The likelihood of developing a food allergy can increase with exposure. For example, rice allergy is more common in East Asia where it forms a large part of the diet, while in Japan, allergy to buckwheat flour, used for soba noodles, is more common.

In general, people with a food allergy are allergic to more than one type of food, such as dairy and eggs, or peanuts and tree nuts. Children in particular are often allergic to several foods, and they sometimes outgrow these allergies.

Allergic Reactions

When you are allergic to a particular food protein, your immune system goes on the attack. Immunoglobulin E (IgE) antibodies recognize the food proteins as foreign and signal the allergy cells to release a variety of chemicals, such as histamine, that cause the symptoms of allergic reaction. Usually coming on quickly, often within minutes or an hour after ingesting the culprit protein, symptoms may include the following:

- Swelling of the eyelids, face, lips, and tongue

- Hives and itching of the mouth, throat, eyes, and skin

- Nausea, vomiting, diarrhea, cramps, and abdominal pain

- Nasal congestion, wheezing, shortness of breath, or difficulty swallowing

During an acute attack, medical attention must be obtained immediately to prevent anaphylaxis, a severe, whole-body allergic reaction that can lead to anaphylactic shock and may result in death. In addition to acute attacks, some people experience chronic symptoms from food allergies including itching and digestive complaints.

Avoidance Therapy

The only way to prevent an allergic reaction to a specific food is through avoidance. Allergy sufferers need to be vigilant, particularly when dining out at restaurants or at the homes of friends or family who may not be aware of the danger. It's imperative to ask about ingredients if you aren't sure. When in doubt, opt for not taking chances. It's equally important to avoid food products that are made with the offending allergen. For example, peanut oil used in cooking must be avoided by peanut allergy sufferers, while dairy in all its forms must be shunned by milk allergy sufferers. Allergens can sometimes also create reactions simply by being airborne—especially milk proteins—so care must be taken as well at childcare centers and schools.

Living with a food allergy can feel restrictive and unfair, but with patience and knowledge you can adapt. Learning to recognize potentially dangerous situations and finding substitute ingredients to use in your favorite foods allows you to enjoy the pleasures of eating without feeling deprived or stressed.

Intolerance vs. Allergy

Having a food intolerance is not a life-threatening condition, but it can certainly make your life frustrating and bothersome. Also called food sensitivity, food intolerance is the inability to properly digest or fully process certain foods, leading sometimes to chronic symptoms and illness. Sometimes the effects are mild, while for some people the effects can be truly painful. Once intolerances are identified and eliminated from your diet, however, the change in how you feel is often immediate.

Food intolerances are much more common than food allergies and are more likely to occur as we age. The most common intolerance is to dairy products, known as lactose intolerance. Lactose is the name of the sugar present in milk, and lactase is the enzyme required to digest lactose. People who are lactose intolerant have fewer lactase enzymes and consequently have difficulty properly digesting foods containing lactose, such as milk, some cheeses, and ice cream. It is also possible to become temporarily lactose intolerant after a GI virus (a quite common condition) or to be born without lactase (quite a rare circumstance). Most of the time, people have varying degrees of lactose intolerance with similarly varying degrees of symptoms.

GI DIDN'T KNOW!

It is actually normal to be lactose intolerant. It's estimated that 70 percent of the world's adult population has difficulty digesting milk and milk products.

Diagnosing Lack of Lactase

Typical symptoms of lactose intolerance include gas, bloating, cramping, and diarrhea. Less common symptoms include nausea and vomiting. These symptoms usually begin shortly after ingesting dairy products but may be delayed up to 24 hours. Because these symptoms are so similar to other GI disorders, it is often difficult to know the cause, but if you are able to document what you have eaten along with any symptoms that arise, you can often make the association on your own.

Sometimes it is helpful to perform a "food challenge" in which you go off dairy foods for a period of time and then reintroduce them into your diet. Keep a food diary to note differences in the way you feel and any specific digestive symptoms that arise. It is also possible to have your doctor perform a breath hydrogen test in which you drink a lactose-containing liquid and then have your breath tested several hours later for the presence of hydrogen, often a tell-tale sign of lactose intolerance. The test is not foolproof, however, so a food diary or challenge may end up being your best means of diagnosis.

Living Lactose Free

Surprisingly, many people with lactase deficiency can usually tolerate small amounts of dairy food, especially as part of a meal, as opposed to drinking a glass of milk on its own. Symptoms can usually be avoided by spreading out the consumption of lactose-rich products over the course of a day, eating or drinking less at any specific meal.

There are dairy products processed with enzymes and labeled "lactose free" that may help some people avoid bothersome symptoms. In a pinch, when a lactose-rich meal cannot be avoided, supplemental lactase enzymes can be taken in either chewable or dissolvable form at the first bite of a meal or drink containing dairy foods.

More Intolerance

Some people cannot tolerate foods containing sugars other than lactose, such as fructose and sorbitol. Gluten may also be a cause for intolerance, separate from celiac disease (see Chapter 8). Less common causes may be foods that contain monosodium glutamate (MSG), *sulfites*, or histamines.

> **DEFINITION**
>
> **Sulfites** are chemical compounds naturally occurring in wine and often used as a preservative in foods including dried fruit, baked goods, condiments, and some dairy products.

Fructose is found in many common foods, particularly fruits such as figs, pears, prunes, and grapes. It is also found in corn syrup, which is often used to sweeten foods, gums, candies, and sodas. In people who cannot properly absorb fructose, symptoms similar to lactose intolerance occur. Sugarless or diet foods, beverages, and even some low-calorie gums are sweetened with sugars that are poorly absorbed by most people. If enough of these foods or beverages are ingested, the load of nonabsorbed sugar that reaches the large intestine can again cause symptoms similar to those of lactose intolerance. Sorbitol, mannitol, and xylitol are a few of the words to look for on labels.

The Bottom Line

By far, the best way to determine whether you have a problem with certain foods is to keep a food diary, including notations on what, when, where, and how you were eating. This type of information is valuable to your doctor when you discuss your symptoms and plays a big part in your diagnosis. In addition, any symptoms that you think are simply the result of a food intolerance should nevertheless be brought to your doctor's attention. There may indeed be another, more serious cause for which you should be tested.

Common Restricted or Special Diets

On occasion it may be necessary to eliminate certain foods from your diet under doctor's orders. This step might be preparation for testing, for healing after an acute attack or surgery, or as part of a long-term program in order to improve your digestive health. When specific diets are required, your doctor often provides you with a set of instructions or refers you to a dietitian. Still, it's worthwhile knowing what to expect if a restricted or special diet is in your future so you can prepare yourself and alert family and friends to specific rules you must follow. The following are a few of the more common diets prescribed for GI conditions.

High Fiber

A high-fiber diet causes a large, soft, bulky stool that passes through the bowel easily and quickly. Because of this action, some digestive tract disorders may be avoided, halted, or even reversed. A softer, larger stool helps prevent constipation and straining. It can also avoid or relieve hemorrhoids. More bulk means less pressure in the colon, which is important in the treatment of IBS and diverticulosis.

The key is to get a good balance of insoluble as well as soluble fiber. Try to consume 35 grams of fiber per day, perhaps even more if your doctor or dietitian recommends you do so. Including the following foods in your diet will help you reach that goal.

Insoluble fiber	Whole-wheat bread and baked goods
	Wheat bran
	Whole-grain breads
	Vegetables and fruit, especially skins
	Peanuts
	Brazil nuts
	Popcorn
	Brown rice and other whole grains
Soluble fiber	Oats in any form (cereals and muffins)
	Apples, oranges, grapefruit, peaches, prunes, pears, and cranberries
	Beans of all kinds
	Beets
	Carrots
	Psyllium or flaxseed meal

Be sure to drink plenty of water throughout the day. If you are not used to eating a good amount of fiber, you may initially experience gas and bloating and may want to speak to your doctor about working more slowly toward your high-fiber goals.

Low Residue/Low Fiber

A low-*residue*/low-fiber diet may be recommended during the flare-up periods of diverticulitis and IBD, including Crohn's and ulcerative colitis (UC). Such a diet may also be recommended as a pre- and post-operation diet to decrease bowel volume.

An intake of less than 10 grams of fiber per day is generally considered low enough, but always check with your doctor.

> **DEFINITION**
>
> **Residue** is the medical term used to describe the solid contents that have reached the lower intestine after most digestion has taken place.

Many people use the terms *low-residue diet* and *low-fiber diet* interchangeably, but in actuality they are not exactly the same. Some low-fiber foods, such as dairy products and coffee, can actually increase residue or stimulate bowel movement. In addition, some foods that are lower in residue, such as bran, are indeed high in fiber. In general, a low-residue diet is for a short time and is more restrictive, so be sure to speak with your doctor if it is required and ask whether he or she suggests that you take vitamin supplements during this period.

Grain products	Enriched, refined white bread and buns, bagels, and English muffins Plain cereals such as Cheerios, corn flakes, Cream of Wheat, Rice Krispies, and Special K Arrowroot cookies, tea biscuits, soda crackers, and plain melba toast White rice and refined pasta and noodles *Avoid whole grains*
Fruits	Fruit juices except prune juice Applesauce and cooked apricots Cantaloupe, honeydew melon, and watermelon *Avoid dried fruits, raisins, and berries*
Vegetables	Vegetable juices Potatoes (no skin) Well-cooked, tender vegetables including beets, green beans, carrots, celery, eggplant, lettuce, mushrooms, green or red peppers, squash, and zucchini *Avoid vegetables from the cruciferous family including broccoli, cauliflower, Brussels sprouts, cabbage, kale, and chard* *Avoid beans, lentils, and other legumes*
Meats	Well-cooked, tender meats; fish; and eggs

In addition, avoid all nuts and seeds, as well as foods that may contain seeds such as breads or whole fruit yogurt. Check with your doctor regarding dairy recommendations.

Clear Liquid

A diet of clear liquids maintains vital body fluids, salts, and minerals, as well as providing at least some energy for patients when normal food intake must be interrupted. Clear liquids are easily absorbed by the body and reduce stimulation of the digestive system, leaving no residue in the intestinal tract. For this reason, a clear liquid diet is often prescribed in preparation for surgery and is generally the first diet given by mouth after surgery. Clear liquids are also given when a person has been without food by mouth (NPO) for a long time. This diet is also often used in preparation for medical tests such as sigmoidoscopy, colonoscopy, or certain x-rays.

Allowed	Fruit juices without pulp
	Gelatin, fruit ice, and popsicle without pulp
	Clear hard candy
	Coffee, tea, soft drinks, and water
	Bouillon, broth, and consommé (fat free)

Low Fat

For a regular healthy diet, no more than 30 percent of total calories should come from fat. However, certain diseases and conditions make it difficult for the body to tolerate much fat at all, in which case a low-fat diet may be recommended. For example, when gallstones or gallbladder disease is present, a low-fat diet is often used to prevent complications. If delayed stomach emptying (gastroparesis) is a problem—often seen in diabetics—a low-fat diet may be helpful. Fat in foods delays stomach emptying, making gastroparesis worse. Other conditions for which a low-fat diet may be beneficial include diarrhea, fatty liver, or obesity.

Although there are any number of low-fat diets you can follow, here are some ways you can easily reduce the amount of fat in your food:

- Use nonstick cooking spray instead of butter or oil.
- Select extra-lean meat and skinless chicken breasts.

- Always trim all visible fat from meats before cooking.

- Avoid frying and opt for baking, broiling, or grilling.

- Drain fat from cooked stews and soups.

- Substitute turkey bacon for regular bacon.

- Eat at least two fish dishes per week.

- Eat at least one vegetarian dish per week.

- Use fat-free broth for gravies and soups.

- Substitute reduced-fat dairy products for full-fat ones.

Low Protein

Low-protein diets are used routinely to treat patients with liver disease, kidney failure, and disorders involving the urea cycle, the metabolism, and amino acids. They are generally meant to reduce the workload of the liver and/or kidneys while providing adequate nutrition. Usually, serious liver and kidney disease are accompanied by the need to limit sodium intake due to high blood pressure or fluid retention. Consequently, table salt (the primary source of sodium in the diet), along with other foods with high sodium content, usually needs to be limited as well. You should not undertake this type of diet on your own. A registered dietitian can help you formulate an appropriate meal plan under the supervision of your doctor.

The Least You Need to Know

- Food allergies involve the immune system and can cause serious allergic symptoms, requiring strict avoidance.

- Common food allergies are dairy, eggs, peanuts, tree nuts, shellfish, seafood, soy, and wheat, with sesame seeds sometimes included.

- Food intolerances are not as serious as food allergies and do not involve the immune system. Rather, they are an inability or reduced ability to digest specific foods.

- Lactose intolerance is the most common type of food intolerance and can be easily managed.

- Occasionally restricted diets are necessary to follow before testing, after surgery, or during healing from a digestive disease, and should be undertaken with the supervision of your doctor or a dietitian.
- Common restricted diets include low residue/low fiber, clear liquid, low fat, and low protein. High-fiber diets are also often recommended.

Natural Remedies and Complementary Therapies

In This Chapter

- Incorporating alternative methods of healing
- Nature's medicine cabinet
- Beneficial therapeutic techniques

The ancient Greek physician Hippocrates said to "let food be thy medicine." His remark wasn't merely a guess that many foods had the ability to heal; it came from years of experience and many cases he saw as a doctor. Of course, Hippocrates was working centuries before synthetic pharmaceuticals, and natural remedies were usually the only ones available, many of them coming from food used on a regular basis. Although many concoctions have since proved invalid—saffron, walnuts, and honey cannot cure the plague—some remedies have managed to survive the test of time and even today can be helpful in coping with minor digestive symptoms.

In this chapter, we'll take a look at some of Mother Nature's resources that may be beneficial in alleviating and even preventing some common symptoms and conditions. Although not recommended as a replacement for medical attention and prescribed medication, a few of these natural ingredients kept on hand might prove helpful when minor tummy upsets or morning sickness arises.

We'll also look at some popular, reputable complementary therapies that, when combined with traditional approaches to medicine, can increase the possibility of recovery from certain conditions such as irritable bowel syndrome (IBS). These healing therapies can sometimes fit into a solid program of maintaining or improving your digestive health.

Nature's Way

People all over the world have incorporated the healing properties of specific foods into their diet for centuries with excellent results. Unfortunately, there have been only a limited number of truly scientific studies on the subject. Recently, however, consumers have become more interested in alternative methods of healing. Many patients ask their doctors whether there is a natural remedy available for their illnesses or whether there is something they can add to their diet to help combat uncomfortable symptoms. The more studies that are conducted, the better equipped doctors become to answer these questions. The study of *functional food* is on the rise in the field of food science and will find its place in the field of modern medicine. For now, here are some natural ways you can contribute to your digestive as well as overall health and remedy some common ailments.

> **DEFINITION**
>
> **Functional food** is any food that may have a health-promoting or disease-preventing property beyond the basic function of supplying nutrients. For example, fermented foods such as yogurt with live cultures are functional foods because in addition to containing vitamins and minerals, they carry probiotic benefits.

Apples

It just may be true: an apple a day could keep the doctor away, including the gastro-enterologist. Research conducted at Sammons Cancer Center in Dallas found that the annurca variety of apple from southern Italy is rich in polyphenols associated with cancer prevention. The incidence of colon cancer is lower in southern Italy than anywhere else in the Western world.

All varieties of apples, however, are an excellent source of dietary fiber, particularly pectin, a type of soluble fiber, as well as vitamin C, potassium, and quercetin, a potent antioxidant. Eating the peel as well as the fruit itself increases the apple's health-related benefits by doing the following:

- Lowering cholesterol
- Reducing inflammation
- Encouraging regular bowel movements

Artichokes

The globe artichoke is one of the oldest known cultivated vegetables, originating from Ethiopia, with Italy currently being the world's largest producer. French and Spanish explorers first brought artichokes to the shores of America, and today virtually all of the globe artichokes produced in the United States grow near Castroville, California.

Artichokes are an excellent source of dietary fiber, magnesium, and the trace mineral chromium. They also contain good amounts of vitamin C, folic acid, biotin, and several B vitamins, including niacin. It is a particularly good source of prebiotics in the form of inulin, which helps to feed friendly bacteria in the gut. Some studies have shown that artichokes may hold other health benefits as well, including the following:

- Lowering cholesterol
- Promoting bile secretion
- Alleviating dyspepsia
- Relieving IBS symptoms

GI DIDN'T KNOW!

Ancient Greeks and Romans valued artichokes as a digestive aid. Because they were scarce, artichokes were available only to the wealthy, who offered them at the end of lavish meals to provide relief from overeating and indigestion.

Avocados

Avocados, originating in Mexico, were introduced into Jamaica in the 1800s, and cultivation in the United States began in 1871 with trees from Mexico. Today Mexico is still the top producer, but the United States and Brazil are not far behind.

Once upon a time, avocados were considered taboo for dieters, diabetics, and heart patients because of their high fat content. But studies have since shown that the type of fat avocados contain, the monounsaturated variety, is actually good for health. In addition to containing "good" fat, avocados are an excellent source of soluble fiber, folate (for cell growth), vitamin B_6, and potassium, as well as the antioxidant vitamins C and E.

A 2000 study in Honolulu discovered that avocados contain potent phytochemicals that may reduce liver damage and could be particularly promising for the treatment of viral hepatitis. Other health benefits may include the following:

- Raising good cholesterol
- Lowering triglycerides
- Promoting skin health
- Improving glucose control

Bananas

Bananas originated in Malaysia 4,000 years ago and were first introduced into Africa before Portuguese explorers took them to the Americas in the late fifteenth century. Since then, bananas have become the second largest fruit crop in the world, and for good reason.

An excellent source of potassium, vitamin B_6, vitamin C, and riboflavin, bananas have long been used to combat diarrhea and are an excellent source of the prebiotic fructooligosaccharide (see Chapter 16). With its high pectin content, the banana is also a good source of soluble fiber and contributes to bowel regularity. Some other health benefits may include the following:

- Regulating blood pressure
- Treating constipation and diarrhea
- Fighting *H. pylori* bacteria

Blueberries

The blueberry is native to North America, and there is some evidence to suggest that humans have consumed blueberries since prehistoric times. Commercial cultivation began in the early 1900s in New Jersey, and today the United States is the largest producer of blueberries in the world.

Although an excellent source of vitamin C, blueberries are particularly prized for their anthocyandins—potent antioxidants—that are responsible for the blueberries' pigment. In a study of 60 fruits and vegetables, the antioxidant capabilities of blueberries rated highest. In studies at the Montreal Diabetes Research Center, extracts of blueberries show promise for use as a complementary antidiabetic therapy. Other health benefits may include the following:

- Reducing the risk of Alzheimer's disease

- Preventing urinary tract infections

- Fighting free radical damage

Broccoli

A member of the cruciferous family and abundant for centuries worldwide, broccoli—once called "Italian asparagus"—became a popular addition to American cuisine only in the 1920s. Since then, its contribution to healthy eating has grown considerably. Broccoli is an excellent source of vitamins K, C, and A; folic acid; and dietary fiber. It's also a good source of phosphorus, potassium, magnesium, and vitamins B_6 and E.

Today, there is much focus on broccoli sprouts, the small alfalfa sprout–looking tender shoots that are eaten raw in salads and sandwiches. They contain extremely high concentrations of sulphoraphane, a phytochemical believed to have great anticarcinogenic promise, among other worthwhile health properties, including the following:

- Fighting *H. pylori* bacteria

- Reducing gastrointestinal cancers

- Reducing breast cancer risk

Cabbage

Although not everyone's favorite vegetable, cabbage and its many varieties should surely be on a list of healthy, healing foods. Also part of the cruciferous family that includes broccoli, cabbage and its antioxidant properties are being explored as potential ways to fight disease.

A particularly good source of vitamin C, potassium, folic acid, vitamin B_6, biotin, calcium, and magnesium, cabbage also contains glucosinolates, which are important phytochemicals that may improve the body's ability to detoxify. Cabbage also contains glutamine, an amino acid with anti-inflammatory properties. Research at the Stanford University School of Medicine demonstrated that fresh cabbage juice is extremely effective in the treatment of peptic ulcers, thanks to its high levels of glutamine. Other healing properties of cabbage may include the following on the next page.

- Regulating the immune system

- Improving intestinal health and regularity

- Reducing bladder cancer risk

> **GI DIDN'T KNOW!**
>
> In the oldest surviving work of Latin prose, *De agri cultura* (*On Farming*), the author, Cato the Elder, remarks on the medicinal values of cabbage.

Flaxseed

Hippocrates, the ancient Greek physician, promoted the use of flax for the relief of abdominal pains. Charlemagne, King of the Franks and ruler of Western Europe in the ninth century, declared the consumption of flax compulsory for his subjects to promote good health. These unusual seeds, first introduced into the United States by early colonists, have received most of their attention because of the omega-3 fatty acids they contain (see Chapter 16). But flaxseeds may hold even more value.

In a double-blind study, 55 people with chronic constipation caused by IBS received either ground flaxseed or psyllium seed daily for three months. Those taking flaxseed had significantly fewer problems with constipation, abdominal pain, and bloating than those taking psyllium. The flaxseed group had even further improvements in constipation and bloating while continuing their treatment in the three months after the double-blind part of the study ended. These results led the researcher to conclude that flaxseed relieved constipation more effectively than psyllium.

The fiber in flaxseed binds with water, swelling to form a gel that, like other forms of fiber, helps soften the stool and move it along in the intestines. In Germany, the Health Commission authorizes the use of flaxseed for various digestive problems such as chronic constipation, IBS, diverticular disease, and general stomach discomfort. Other benefits may include the following:

- Reducing prostate and breast cancer risk

- Lowering cholesterol

- Reducing inflammation

Garlic

The therapeutic uses of garlic date back to ancient Egyptian times and were particularly popular in Greek and Roman medicine. Prized as an effective remedy for a variety of ailments, garlic's antibacterial properties in particular were explored by the microbiologist Louis Pasteur in the nineteenth century.

An excellent source of vitamin B_6, garlic also contains a good amount of manganese, selenium, and vitamin C. Allicin, however, is the chemical compound that gives garlic its antimicrobial and antifungal properties as well as its distinctive odor. In a promising preliminary study, allicin showed significant antibacterial activity against drug-resistant *Shigella dysenteriae*, the bacteria that causes the most severe dysentery. Further research is required, however, to determine the effectiveness of garlic and its allicin in the general treatment of dysentery.

In an observational four-year trial involving 41,837 women, results showed that women whose diets included significant quantities of garlic were approximately 30 percent less likely to develop colon cancer. Although more scientific study needs to be conducted, garlic clearly shows great promise as a healing, functional food for the digestive system. Its other benefits may include the following:

- Lowering bad cholesterol
- Raising good cholesterol
- Treating fungal skin infections
- Reducing the risk and severity of common colds

Ginger

The medicinal properties of ginger have been known for centuries. Chinese cooks have added ginger to dishes not only for its intense flavor but to counter the effects of potential toxins in animal protein and to stimulate digestion. The ancient Greeks used ginger's ability to counteract vertigo and motion sickness. During the Middle Ages, ginger was thought to remedy the plague and, in the form of gingerbread, provide strength for knights going into battle.

TUMMY TIP

Many moms-to-be find that ginger lollipops can relieve pregnancy-related nausea.

Today, the healing nature of ginger is recognized for its anti-inflammatory properties in the treatment of arthritis and bursitis and as a remedy for nausea and menstrual cramps. Gingerol is the potent antioxidant it contains that can reduce inflammation and pain in much the same way nonsteroidal anti-inflammatory drugs (NSAIDs) do, but without the undesirable side effects. Other potential benefits are as follows:

- Inhibiting *H. pylori* bacteria growth

- Treating motion sickness

- Reducing pain from inflammation

Peppermint

Historically, peppermint has been used medicinally as a general digestive aid and for the symptomatic treatment of upper respiratory infections. Peppermint oil has shown to be particularly good as a natural antispasmodic, relieving muscle contractions in the digestive tract.

GULP!

If you suffer from acid reflux disease or have heartburn associated with dyspepsia, peppermint may not be for you. It relaxes the lower esophageal sphincter (LES), allowing acid to backwash into the throat.

In a one-month double-blind, placebo-controlled clinical study involving 110 participants with symptoms of IBS, there was significant improvement of symptoms after taking a peppermint oil formulation three to four times daily. In another study, 57 participants took peppermint oil capsules twice daily for four weeks, and 75 percent of them showed a 50 percent decrease of IBS symptoms. Peppermint oil may also be effective in the following:

- Reducing indigestion

- Treating fungus infections

- Reducing tension headaches

Tea

Did you know that drinking just two cups of tea a day could increase your antioxidant levels? Studies have shown that tea polyphenols have a great capacity to prevent free radicals from harming cells and may even protect against heart disease by inhibiting blood platelets from clumping together. Green tea, oolong tea, and black tea are all protective, whether decaffeinated or not, but green tea, because of its unique processing, appears to offer the greatest benefits.

Green tea originates from China and is also now cultivated in India, Sri Lanka (Ceylon), and Japan. In the United States, consumption of green tea has increased dramatically since its association with good health. Green tea has, in fact, been proven to reduce the risk of gastric cancer in women. Other benefits may include the following:

- Reducing the risk of type 2 diabetes
- Reducing tooth decay
- Assisting in weight loss

TUMMY TIP

A specific type of Japanese green tea called kukicha twig tea may help dieters. It is particularly bitter and believed to balance the body's desire for sugary substances. Western palates tend to avoid bitter tastes, preferring instead the sensations of salt, sour, sweet, and pungent. Increasing the bitter taste sensation in your diet might lessen your desire for sugary treats.

Complementary Therapies

Complementary therapies are forms of *alternative medicine* that, when used alongside traditional approaches, assist in treating particular diseases and conditions. Common alternative medicine practices include naturopathy, chiropractic, herbalism, traditional Chinese medicine, Ayurveda, meditation, yoga, biofeedback, hypnosis, homeopathy, acupuncture, and diet-based therapies.

DEFINITION

Alternative medicine is any healing practice that does not fall within the realm of conventional Western medicine and that may not have a body of scientific evidence in support of its approach.

Relaxation-promoting therapies are usually grouped under the term cognitive behavioral therapy (CBT), and studies have shown that in patients with many simultaneous pain syndromes such as IBS, fibromyalgia, migraine headaches, chronic interstitial cystitis, and chronic fatigue syndrome, outcomes are better with these approaches than with medication. Although not all alternative approaches have been used with conventional medicine in a complementary sense, many have. Here are just a few that have shown promise in treating digestive disorders in conjunction with mainstream approaches.

Acupuncture

A form of Traditional Chinese Medicine (TCM), acupuncture is the procedure of inserting and manipulating fine, threadlike needles into specific points on the body to relieve pain or provide therapy. It is based on the concept of qi or ch'i, the vital energy that some philosophies assert flows through us. Practitioners target particular acupuncture points or meridians that are thought to be related to specific parts of the body. By stimulating these points, the intention is to adjust the energy flow so the body can heal itself.

Acupuncture has been the subject of active scientific research since the late twentieth century, but it still remains controversial. The World Health Organization published a review of controlled trials using acupuncture and concluded it was effective for the treatment of 28 conditions, while the American Academy of Medical Acupuncture has pointed to a number of conditions and diseases that could be addressed with acupuncture as a complementary therapy, including the following:

- Abdominal distention or flatulence
- Acute and chronic pain control
- Constipation and diarrhea
- Nausea and vomiting
- Acid reflux
- IBS

Hypnotherapy

Hypnotherapy uses hypnosis, a mental state induced by instructions and suggestions, to attempt to modify a person's behavior, emotional content, and attitudes. Hypnotherapists also address a wide range of conditions, including dysfunctional habits, anxiety, stress-related illness, pain management, and personal development. A hypnotherapist differs from other therapists by focusing on the role of subconscious behaviors and influences on a client's life.

GI DIDN'T KNOW!

During the mid-nineteenth century, hypnosis was used to alleviate pain and distress during surgery. The founder of hypnotherapy, James Braid, was a surgeon himself specializing in muscular conditions, and he reported many cases of minor surgery using hypnotism.

In 1999, the *British Medical Journal* (*BMJ*) published a review of current medical research on hypnotherapy and relaxation therapies, finding sufficient evidence that these therapies were valid for treating a number of conditions. Since then, numerous reports have indicated there is convincing evidence that clinical hypnotherapy is effective in treating the following:

- Acute and chronic pain
- Anxiety and stress
- Headaches and migraines
- IBS

Meditation

A mental discipline practiced since antiquity, meditation attempts to take the mind into a deeper state of relaxation or awareness. It often involves turning your attention to a single point of reference through visualizing a place or thing or by focusing on your breath. Different meditative disciplines encompass a wide range of spiritual or psychophysical practices that may emphasize different goals, from achievement of a higher state of consciousness to greater focus, creativity, or self-awareness or simply a more relaxed and peaceful frame of mind.

Meditation has entered the mainstream of health care as a method of stress and pain reduction. In an early study in 1972, meditation was shown to reduce byproducts of stress such as lactate, decrease heart rate and blood pressure, and induce favorable brain waves. Since then, this "relaxation response" and accompanying brain activity has been confirmed by functional MRI imaging that measures blood flow to the brain. Although its actual effect on disease is difficult to evaluate, as a relaxation technique, meditation is a valuable complementary tool for digestive disorders such as IBS and those requiring pain management.

Qigong

An internal Chinese meditative practice, qigong (or ch'i kung) uses slow graceful movements and controlled breathing techniques to promote the circulation of qi within the human body and to enhance overall health. Some Western medical practitioners believe it has possible benefits to health through stress reduction and exercise. Many patients have testified to a reduction or elimination of pain through its practice. Qigong can be performed while perfectly still as well as with movement or while seated comfortably, which makes it an ideal complementary therapy when patients are less than mobile.

In 2009, a randomized clinical trial on cancer patients concluded that medical qigong, along with conventional health care, can improve overall quality of life, fatigue, and positive mood status and reduce the side effects of nausea, sleep disturbance, and inflammation. It may also improve digestion through posture and stretching.

Tai Chi

Also known as t'ai chi ch'uan, this type of internal Chinese martial art is often practiced for health reasons. Popular worldwide, medical studies of tai chi support its effectiveness as an alternative exercise and a form of martial arts therapy. By focusing the mind solely on the movements of the body, tai chi is believed to help bring about a state of mental calm and clarity. Tai chi classes have become popular in hospitals and clinics, as well as community and senior centers, in the last 20 years or so as its reputation as a form of low-stress training for seniors has become better known.

Tai chi is in the process of being subjected to rigorous scientific studies in the West in order to determine what style and duration is most beneficial as a form of exercise. In addition to improved balance and flexibility, possible strengthening of the immune system and reduced severity of diabetes are potential benefits being currently examined. In the meantime, as a light form of exercise (especially for seniors) and as a stress-relieving and relaxing activity, tai chi may be helpful to a number of people with chronic digestive conditions, including IBS.

Yoga

Yoga is a healing system of theory and practice using a combination of breathing exercises, physical postures, and meditation that has been practiced for more than 5,000 years. Although developed as a spiritual practice in the East, yoga's popularity in the West has focused primarily on the physical exercise aspect. However, as interest in yoga has grown since its introduction to the United States in the nineteenth century, it is considered by many to be a mind-body intervention useful in reducing the health effects of generalized stress.

GI DIDN'T KNOW!

It's estimated that 30 million Americans practice some form of yoga on a regular basis.

Most beginning yoga classes consist of a gentle combination of physical exercises, breathing exercises, and meditation. These characteristics make yoga a particularly beneficial kind of exercise for people with certain health conditions, including heart disease, hypertension, asthma, back problems, and digestive disorders, particularly related to constipation and regularity.

The Least You Need to Know

- Many remedies for common digestive symptoms can be found in nature, particularly in the food we eat.
- Green tea, ginger, and peppermint have been proven to be beneficial for some digestive health problems while also being preventive in nature.
- Complementary therapies are alternative approaches that are used in conjunction with mainstream medicine.
- Relaxation therapies have been shown to be particularly helpful for conditions such as IBS.
- Continuing studies on the use of complementary approaches with conventional medicine are being done in order to optimize patient outcomes.

Glossary

abdomen   The area between the chest and the hips that contains the stomach, small intestine, large intestine, liver, gallbladder, pancreas, and spleen.

achalasia   Death of inhibitory cells of the esophagus causing the failure of the lower esophageal sphincter, a valve that separates the stomach and the esophagus, to open.

acute   Sudden onset of symptoms.

aerophagia   Ingestion of air.

amino acids   A group of 20 different kinds of small molecules that link in long chains to form proteins.

anal fissure   A cut in the anal canal.

anastomosis, intestinal   Reattachment of two portions of bowel.

antispasmodics   Drugs that inhibit smooth muscle contraction in the gastrointestinal tract.

anus   The opening of the rectum.

autonomic nervous system   The part of the nervous system that controls involuntary actions of internal organs such as the bowel.

barium   A metallic, chemical, chalky liquid used to coat the inside of organs so that they will show up on an x-ray.

bile   Secretions of the liver that aid in digestion and absorption and that stimulate peristalsis.

biliary tract   The gallbladder and the bile ducts.

biopsy   A tissue sample.

borborygmi   Audible, rumbling abdominal sounds due to gas gurgling with liquid as it passes through the intestines.

bowel   The intestines.

brain-belly connection   The continuous back and forth exchange of information and feedback that takes place between the gastrointestinal tract and the brain and spinal cord.

capsule endoscopy   A procedure that lets your doctor examine the lining of the middle part of your gastrointestinal tract by using a pill-size video capsule that you swallow.

celiac disease   An allergic reaction of the lining of the small intestine in response to the protein gliadin (a component of gluten). Gliadin is found in wheat, rye, barley, and oats. Celiac disease is also called celiac sprue or gluten intolerance.

chronic   Symptoms occurring over a long period of time.

***Clostridium difficile* (*C. difficile*)**   A gram-positive anaerobic bacterium. *C. difficile* is recognized as the major causative agent of colitis (inflammation of the colon) and diarrhea that may occur following antibiotic intake.

colectomy   Removal of part or all of the colon.

colitis   Inflammation of the colon.

colon   The large intestine.

colonoscopy   A fiberoptic (endoscopic) procedure in which a thin, flexible, lighted viewing tube (a colonoscope) is threaded up through the rectum for the purpose of inspecting the entire colon and rectum and, if there is an abnormality, taking a tissue sample of it (biopsy) for examination under a microscope, or removing it.

colostomy   A surgically created opening of the colon to the abdominal wall, allowing the diversion of fecal waste.

congenital   A condition existing at birth but not through heredity.

constipation   Reduced stool frequency, hard stools, difficulty passing stools, or painful bowel movements.

contrast radiology   A test in which a contrast material (such as barium) is used to coat the rectum, colon, and lower part of the small intestine so they show up on an x-ray.

Crohn's disease (CD)   A form of inflammatory bowel disease.

dehydration   An excessive loss of fluids in the body.

diabetes A disease in which blood glucose (blood sugar) levels are above normal. Type 2 diabetes, also known as adult-onset or noninsulin-dependent diabetes mellitus, is the most common form of diabetes.

diaphragm The muscle wall between the chest and the abdomen.

diarrhea Passing frequent and loose stools that can be watery. Acute diarrhea goes away in a few weeks and becomes chronic when it lasts longer than four weeks.

dilatation Expansion of an organ or vessel; dilation.

disorder A disturbance in regular or normal function; an abnormal condition.

distention A swelling of the abdomen.

diverticula (diverticulosis) Small pouches in the colon.

diverticulitis A condition that occurs when a diverticulum becomes infected or irritated.

duodenum The first part of the small intestine.

dysphagia The sensation of food sticking in the esophagus.

electrolytes Chemicals that break down into ions (atoms) in the body's fluids and are essential to regulating many body functions.

endoscope A thin, flexible tube with a light and a lens on the end used to look into the esophagus, stomach, duodenum, small intestine, colon, or rectum.

endoscopy A procedure that uses an endoscope to diagnose or treat a condition. There are many types of endoscopy; examples include colonoscopy, sigmoidoscopy, gastroscopy, enteroscopy, and esophogogastroduodenoscopy.

enteral nutrition Food provided through a tube placed in the nose, stomach, or small intestine.

enteric nervous system (ENS) Autonomic nervous system within the walls of the digestive tract. The ENS regulates digestion and the muscle contractions that eliminate solid waste.

enteritis An irritation of the small intestine.

enterocolitis Inflammation of the intestinal ganglion; a mass of nerve cells.

enteroscopy Examination of the inside of the small intestine using an endoscope.

eosinophilic gastroenteritis   A rare disease characterized by food-related reactions, infiltration of certain white blood cells (eosinophils) in the GI tract, and an increase in the number of eosinophils in the blood.

esophagitis   An irritation of the esophagus.

esophagogastroduodenoscopy (EGD)   Examination of the inside of the esophagus, stomach, and duodenum using an endoscope.

esophagus   The organ that connects the mouth to the stomach.

familial   Tending to occur in more members of a family than expected by chance alone.

feces   Waste eliminated from the bowels.

fistula   An abnormal passage between two organs or between an organ and the outside of the body.

food allergy   An immune system response by which the body creates antibodies as a reaction to certain food.

functional disorder   A disorder or disease in which the primary abnormality is an alteration in the way the body works (physiological function). It characterizes a disorder that generally cannot be diagnosed in a traditional way.

gastric   Related to the stomach.

gastric juices   Liquids produced in the stomach to help break down food and kill bacteria.

gastritis   An inflammation of the stomach lining.

gastroenteritis   An infection or irritation of the stomach and intestines.

gastroenterologist   A doctor who specializes in digestive diseases or disorders.

gastroenterology   The field of medicine concerned with the function and disorders of the digestive system.

gastroesophageal reflux disease (GERD)   Also called acid reflux, a condition in which the contents of the stomach regurgitate (or back up) into the esophagus (food pipe), causing discomfort and sometimes esophageal injury.

gastrointestinal (GI) tract   The muscular tube from the mouth to the anus, also called the alimentary canal or digestive tract.

gastroparesis   Nerve or muscle damage in the stomach leading to delayed gastric emptying.

gastroscopy   The examination of the inside of the esophagus, stomach, and duodenum using an endoscope.

gastrostomy (G-tube)   A method of enteral feeding in which a tube is surgically or endoscopically introduced through the abdominal wall.

genome   The complete genetic material of an organism.

H-2 blockers   A class of medicines that reduce the amount of acid the stomach produces.

Helicobacter pylori (*H. pylori*)   A bacterium that can damage stomach and duodenal tissue, causing ulcers and stomach cancer.

hemorrhoids   Veins around or inside the anus or lower rectum that are swollen and inflamed.

hepatic   Related to the liver.

hepatitis   Inflammation of the liver.

hereditary   Genetically transmitted or transmittable from parent to offspring.

hiatal hernia   A small opening in the diaphragm that allows a part of the stomach to move up into the chest.

ileostomy   A surgically created opening of the abdominal wall to the ileum, allowing the diversion of fecal waste.

ileum   The lower third of the small intestine, adjoining the colon.

imaging   Tests that produce pictures of areas inside the body.

imperforate anus   A birth defect in which the anal canal fails to develop. This is treated surgically.

inflammation   Redness, swelling, pain, and/or a feeling of heat in an area of the body. This is a protective reaction to injury, disease, or irritation of the tissues.

inflammatory bowel disease (IBD)   A set of chronic diseases characterized by inflammation, irritation, and ulcers in the gastrointestinal tract. The most common disorders are ulcerative colitis and Crohn's disease.

ingestion   Taking into the body by mouth.

intestinal mucosa   The surface lining of the intestines where the cells absorb nutrients.

intestinal pseudo-obstruction   Symptoms and signs of intestinal blockage but no actual blockage.

intestines   Also known as the bowels or the long, tubelike organs in the human body that complete digestion or the breaking down of food. They consist of the small intestine and the large intestine.

ischemic colitis   Colitis caused by decreased blood flow to the colon.

lactose   A sugar found commonly in milk and dairy products.

lactose intolerance   The inability to digest or absorb lactose.

laparoscopy   The insertion of a thin, lighted tube (called a laparoscope) through the abdominal wall to inspect the inside of the abdomen and remove tissue samples.

large intestine   The long, tubelike organ that is connected to the small intestine at one end and the anus at the other. The large intestine has four parts: cecum, colon, rectum, and anal canal.

manometry   A test that measures pressure or contractions in the gastrointestinal tract.

motility   Movement of contents within the gastrointestinal tract.

neural   Having to do with nerves or the nervous system, including the brain and the spinal cord.

neurotransmitter   A chemical in the nervous system that helps transmit messages.

nutrient   A chemical compound (such as protein, fat, carbohydrate, vitamins, or minerals) that makes up foods.

palpation   Examination by pressing on the surface of the body to feel the organs or tissues underneath.

parenteral nutrition   The slow infusion of a solution of nutrients into a vein through a catheter, which is surgically implanted. This may be partial, to supplement food and nutrient intake, or total.

pathology   The study of the fundamental nature, causes, and development of abnormal conditions and the structural and functional changes that result.

pelvic   Having to do with the pelvis (the lower part of the abdomen located between the hip bones).

peptic ulcer   A sore in the lining of the esophagus, stomach, or duodenum, caused most commonly by the bacterium *H. pylori* or use of NSAID medications. An ulcer in the stomach is a gastric ulcer; an ulcer in the duodenum is a duodenal ulcer.

polyp   A benign growth involving the lining of the GI tract (noncancerous tumors or neoplasms). They can occur in several locations in the gastrointestinal tract but are most common in the colon.

primary care physician   A doctor who manages a person's health care over time. A primary care doctor is able to give a wide range of care, including prevention and treatment, and can refer a patient to a specialist.

prokinetic   Drugs that enhance propulsion of contents through the gut.

protein   A large, complex molecule made up of one or more chains of amino acids. Proteins perform a wide variety of activities in the cell.

proton pump inhibitor (PPI)   The strongest class of drugs for inhibiting acid secretion in the stomach.

rectum   The lower end of the large intestine, leading to the anus.

refractory   Resistant to treatment.

resection, intestinal   The surgical removal of a diseased portion of the intestines.

sigmoid colon   The S-shaped section of the colon that connects to the rectum.

sigmoidoscopy   Examination of the inside of the sigmoid colon and rectum using an endoscope—a thin, lighted tube (sigmoidoscope).

small intestine   The part of the digestive tract that is located between the stomach and the large intestine.

sphincter   A ring of muscle that opens and closes and acts as a valve in various "check points" of the GI tract.

squamous cell   A flat cell that looks like a fish scale under a microscope. Squamous cells cover internal and external surfaces of the body.

stricture   An abnormal narrowing of a tubular part of the body.

syndrome   A set of symptoms or conditions that occur together and suggest the presence of a certain disease or an increased chance of developing the disease.

systemic   Affecting the entire body.

ulcerative colitis (UC)   A form of inflammatory bowel disease that causes ulcers and inflammation in the inner lining of the colon and rectum.

ultrasound   An imaging method in which high-frequency sound waves are used to outline a part of the body.

upper endoscopy   Examination of the inside of the esophagus, stomach, and duodenum using an endoscope.

upper GI series   X-rays of the esophagus, stomach, and duodenum.

valsalva maneuver   Voluntarily increasing pressure in the abdominal cavity with the diaphragm and abdominal muscles to bear down on the rectum to facilitate defecation.

villi   Tiny, fingerlike projections on the surface of the small intestine that help absorb nutrients.

visceral hypersensitivity   Enhanced perception, or over-responsiveness, within the gut, even to normal events.

American Association for the Study of Liver Diseases

www.aasld.org

An excellent resource for both patients and physicians, with current research information on diagnosis and treatment.

American College of Gastroenterology

www.gi.org

Provides accurate and up-to-date information on digestive health issues as well as useful patient resources.

American Gastroenterological Association

www.gastro.org

The oldest medical-specialty society in the United States, with more than 16,500 physicians and researchers as members.

Andrea's Gluten Free Bakery

www.andreasglutenfree.com

A Saint Louis–based bakery that is a favorite for people suffering from celiac disease and others who must also avoid gluten. Ships anywhere in the United States.

Celiac Disease Foundation

www.celiac.org

Support, information, and assistance for those affected by celiac disease.

Celiac.com

www.celiac.com

A website providing gluten-free diet information and assistance for celiac sufferers.

Clinical Trials

www.clinicaltrials.gov

A searchable database for public use that provides information on current clinical trials and research studies.

Crohn's and Colitis Foundation of America

www.ccfa.org

Dedicated to improving the lives of those who suffer with inflammatory bowel diseases.

Enteral Health and Nutrition

www.enteralhealthandnutrition.com

A Saint Louis–based company started by patients to approach their condition naturally. The website often has free recipes and tips for your gastrointestinal health.

IBS Self Help and Support Group

www.ibsgroup.org

A community for sufferers of irritable bowel syndrome, with dependable education and treatment information.

International Foundation for Functional Gastrointestinal Disorders

http://iffgd.org

A nonprofit organization devoted to education and research, with valuable patient resources for gastrointestinal disorders of all types.

National Heartburn Alliance

www.heartburnalliance.org

Answers to all your heartburn questions and concerns.

Patient Advocate Foundation

www.patientadvocate.org

A national network for access to healthcare as well as education and appeals.

Index